# Female Genital Mutilation in the Middle East

# PLACING OMAN ON THE MAP

Hoda Thabet, Ph.D.    &    Azza al-Kharousi, MD

*Female Genital Mutilation in the Middle East: Placing Oman on the Map*

National and University Library of Iceland
ISBN: 978-9935-9256-2-6

http://is.linkedin.com/in/hodathabet

"Oman is not on the map of countries where female genital mutilation is practised. Neither the United Nations nor international NGOs have taken notice of FGM in the Gulf region – except Yemen. Yet, there are quite a number of reports about its existence in Oman and in most other countries on the Arabian Peninsula, some old from the 1960s, others are medical studies about cysts and other complications"[1].

1 https://stopfgmmiddleeast.wordpress.com/2014/01/31/in-oman-more-than-80-of-women-could-be-mutilated-results-of-a-two-week-field-trip/

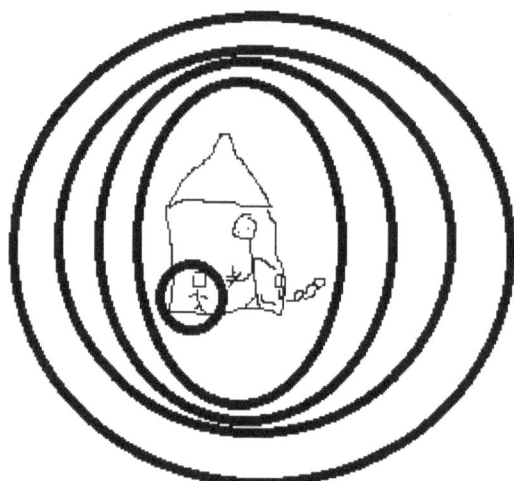

Death

# Acknowledgement

This survey research on the prevalence of female genital mutilation/ cutting practice in Oman is an independent study that has been conducted by two independent researchers. The research team included Azza al-Kharousi, MD and myself, Ph.D.

There were two phases of the research quality management that indicated for conducting this study on the prevalence of FGM/C practice in Oman among the Omani nationals. The first phase included designing the principle research questions. The second phase included collecting data by using the technique of random sampling through conducting a survey with a questionnaire. The survey research involved collecting data from a random sample of adult Omani females who visited a medical clinic in the ad-Dakhiliya province of Oman.

My heartfelt appreciation goes to Azza al-Kharousi, MD. for conducting the field survey at a women health clinic in the ad-Dakhiliya province of Oman. In 1997, Azza al-Kharousi graduated as a Family and Community Medical Doctor from College of Medicine and Health Sciences, Sultan Qaboos University. Currently, she is a Senior Specialist (MRCGP) in Family and Community Medicine, Oman.

*Hoda Thabet, Ph.D*

*Reykjavik- 2018*

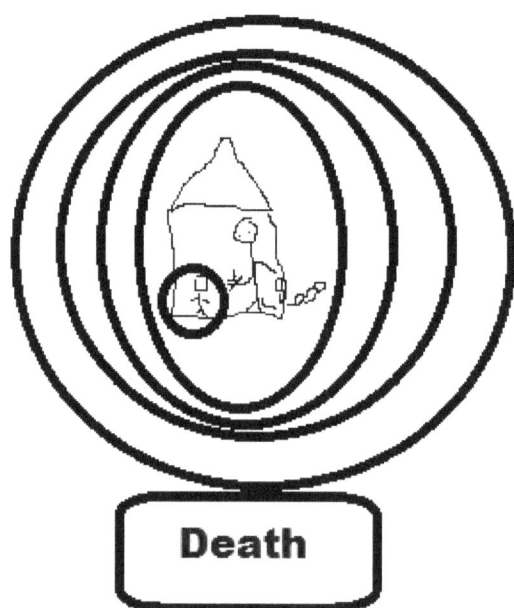

Death

# A note from the field

200 Omani females from various age groups and various educational backgrounds were asked to answer this questionnaire on female genital mutilation in Oman. It was easy to talk about FGM/C to females from the young generation, but many elderly women aged 60 and onwards refused talking about this topic; some of them refused answering the questionnaire. One woman who was in her 70s, started shouting in anger when she was asked about FGM/C. Female gentile mutilation/cutting is not taught in the college of Medicine at Sultan Qaboos university. From the day the college was established in1986 until our present-day, FGM/C is not been included in the study programs and  the medical students do not receive any formal training or education on this subject. During those years that female circumcision was permitted by the government to be performed in Oman's health clinics, the health practitioners were not trained to perform the cutting, as it has never been taught in the college of Medicine. In our present-day, female gentile mutilation/cutting is widely practiced in Oman but it is not permitted by the government. Mostly it is done secretly by  traditional health practitioners. Those traditional health practitioners are old Omani women, and they have not received any medical training to circumcise females.

*Azza al-Kharousi, (MRCGP)*

*Senior Specialist in Family and Community Medicine*

*Oman- 2018*

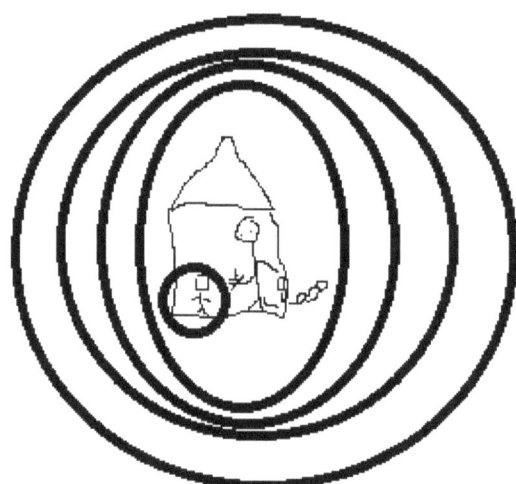

Death

# ABSTRACT

Female genital mutilation/cutting (FGM/C) is a form of gender-based violence that is prevalent among a number of patriarchal cultures across Africa and into the Middle East. Typically practiced on children under the age of ten, it is a violation of human rights that results in serious emotional and physical trauma. To date, the majority of the data available on the topic of FGM/C originates from studies conducted in Africa. While there has been research published regarding FGM/C in the Middle East, the data is sparse. The purpose of this study was to investigate and report upon the prevalence of FGM/C in the Middle Eastern country of Oman and to determine which attributes among the surveyed population were associated with the decision to cut their own daughter(s). Between October and December 2017, 200 females were surveyed at a medical clinic in the ad-Dakhiliya province of Oman. The vast majority of the study population was of Omani descent, married and between the ages of 19 and 45 years old. Importantly, 95.5% of the women surveyed self-reported themselves as having previously undergone FGM/C. Of particular interest is that 86.0% of the study population reported that they planned to—or had already—subjected their daughter(s) to FGM/C. By conducting a chi-square test of independence, it was revealed that variables significantly associated with the decision to cut their daughter(s) were: having undergone FGM/C themselves ($X^2 = 38.60$, p-value<0.05), level of education attained by the study participant ($X^2 = 23.93$, p-value p-value<0.05) and the occupation/employment status of the study participant ($X^2 = 14.05$, p-value<0.05) Age of the participant was not significantly associated with the decision to have FGM/C performed on their daughter(s) ($X^2 = 0.65$, p-value = 0.72). It is hoped that results from this study may help support the creation of recommendations that target the practice of FGM/C in Oman with the intention of increasing awareness and education. Insights gained from this project may also be useful in the creation of new policies at the institutional level condemning FGM/C. The eventual eradication of this horrific and harmful practice is the ultimate goal.

# Female Genital Mutilation
## in the Middle East

# PLACING OMAN
# ON THE MAP

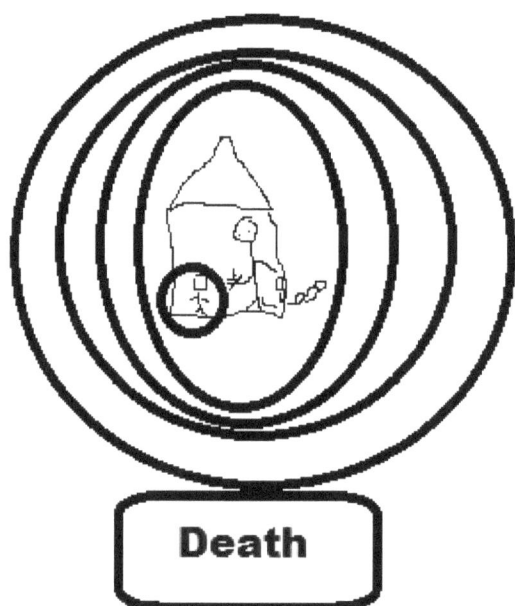

Death

# Table of Contents

# SECTION ONE

## REVIEW OF LITERATURE

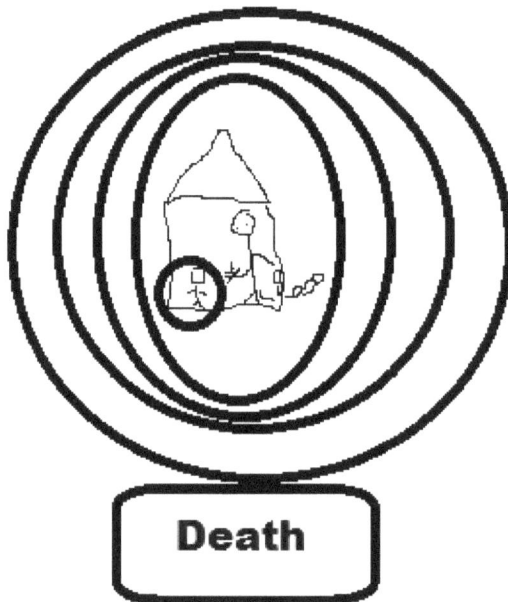

# Chapter One: Introduction

Female genital mutilation FGM/C is a global threat against girls and women and it requires long-lasting global solutions. Research in 2014 revealed that 64% of the Omani female participants have admitted to the practices of FGM/C within their families. The high percentage of these practices questions the widely accepted beliefs at global and regional scale. Because most of the time FGM/C is practiced in secret, the young-girls remain at risk despite the fact that they might be living in countries where FGM/C is prohibited by law. The African Union is a good example, where FGM/C is prohibited by law. FGM/C is practiced widely although in 2016 The African Union approved its abolition in the 50 member states. The practice of FGM/C is closely witnessed in our reality. In Europe, around 180,000 migrant women are annually subjected to FGM/C or at risk of becoming FGM/C.

Mutilation involves the total or partial removal of the female genitalia. It causes physical injuries for life, such as problems during menstruation, difficulties in childbirth, bleeding or infections that sometimes cause the death of the woman and the baby during childbirth. It is usually carried out between childhood and the age of fifteen and is a flagrant violation of the human rights of girls. Almost in majority of cases FGM/C is caused by the widespread rooted traditions and by the community pressure against girls and their families. For example, girls who do not undergo mutilation are considered dirty and men reject marrying them.

Oman has been mentioned in the study of WHO that listed the countries in Africa and Middle East where the practices of FGM/C are being reported. It is evident from the existing literature dedicated towards the study of these practices in Oman that it is widely accepted and followed the practice in the country regardless of prohibited practices in hospitals. Most of the cases remain unreported because they have been carried out by women population of the country within their homes and with willingness. There are various social, cultural and traditional aspects that are worth exploring for the case of Oman to evaluate rationale behind wide acceptance of the practice. Traditional beliefs constructed by the researchers of West lack the wider perspective over inclination of the major population in Oman towards acceptance of FGM/C as normal or mandatory procedure for women. Being an Islamic state there is a possibility of an influence from confused religious stances on the matter.There is no unified state registry of the number of mutilated women and girls living in Oman's territory, which does not allow us to have a clear picture of the prevalence of the phenomenon.

Female genital mutilation constitutes a serious attack against human rights. It is a brutal act of violence that directly affects the physical and psychological integrity of women. Undoubtedly, as established in Article 3 of the European Convention on Human Rights, the mutilation of the genital organs of girls and young women constitutes an "inhuman and degrading" treatment. The practice of totally or partially extirpating the female sex organs has its roots in a totally outdated and radically unjust conception of the place that corresponds to females in a community. In these social structures that are based on unbalanced power relations and in the inequality between the sexes, women occupy a position of inferiority while men exercise a function of dominance over sexuality, autonomy, and their lives. The females, according to an archaic patriarchal concept, would be the depository of the family honour, which would explain the prejudices about their promiscuity and the need of control over their bodies. The social and family pressure suffered by girls is of such magnitude that most do not even conceive of being able to refuse to undergo mutilation. Those who try are marginalized, rejected and isolated from their group. In most cases, little or no training and information about their sexuality makes the victims completely ignorant of the true magnitude of the trauma they will suffer. They only know the physical consequences of mutilation and such vexation "has always existed for women".

In Oman, girls are not recognized as a subject of special protection against genital mutilation. Although the Criminal Code includes the prohibition of genital mutilation or ablation, incorporated as an offence into the legal system, it does not consider that girls deserve special protection. They are hidden under the generic category of "minor", even though they are the ones who suffer the most from genital mutilation. On the occasion of the International Day of Zero Tolerance with Female Genital Mutilation FGM, Plan International, an organization that fights for the rights of children and equality for girls, calls on civil society to become aware and act against a practice that undermines the rights and health of millions of girls around the world. Meanwhile, there is the prevalence of opinion in countries like Oman that certain type of FGM/C is recommendable for young girls and women to acquire a certain level of body cleansing and beauty that is encouraged by the cultures within the country. Regardless of the changing attitude in the country towards modernism and gender, the practice of FGM/C still remains in Oman due to the deviating perspective of the society around it. In order to advocate about this practice which is a globally accepted perception , in the following section we shall explore the gaps between the two opposite perspectives to approach the health care problems associated with FGM/C in Oman.

## 1.2 The rationale behind the prevalence of the practice

The theme of Female Genital Mutilation / Cutting encompasses a wide variety of sub-themes. Before any further development of the subject, it is important that these sub-themes are defined and discussed. According to Amnesty International (1997), FGM/C is the "term used to refer to partial or total removal of female genitalia." However, the term used depends on the country and can also be known as cutting the female genitals. It is a procedure that is divided into four types, ranging from community to community (although not transversal to all) and from country to country. According to Amnesty International (AI), infibulation is the least common type ("about 15% of mutilations in Africa"),–as opposed to clitoridectomy or excision, which account for about 85%–is the more severe. The infibulation, also called Type III, "consists of clitoridectomy (the clitoris is removed totally or partially), excision (total or partial removal of the small lips) and cutting of the large lips" which are then sewn, leaving only a small hole intended for urine output and menstrual blood (Boyle, 2001).

In countries where it is practiced, FGM/C is considered a prerequisite for young females to

21

marry. However, concerning health care of women population, studies have shown that only a limited population in Oman is affected by the physical injuries, such as problems during menstruation, difficulties in childbirth, bleeding or infections. In some part of the country, the men refuse to marry a female who has not been circumcised. Nevertheless, their refusal is rather conveyed secretly as this is considered a hybrid of a woman. Women who are victims of excision have their sexual desire reduced, so that sexual promiscuity also decreases, life without sex becomes more tolerable. Mutilation is thus a certainty as to the fidelity of the bride and the chastity of the bride in certain communities. (Braun, 2010).

FGM/C is a tradition based on misconceptions, there is a belief that the female genitals are "unclean" so that only through extirpation can they be purified. It is also based on the idea that only man has the right to enjoy sexual pleasure. In addition to being discriminatory, this practice is extremely dangerous as it does not involve any hygienic care. The materials used are not sterilized, they are often rusty and it is common to use the same instruments for various excisions (which could lead to the spread of diseases such as AIDS). Among these instruments are knives, pieces of glass, sheets, ice, small tree trunks, thorns, leaves, and herbs. It is therefore very frequent that serious infections occur which, when not leading to death, cause damage to the reproductive health, resulting in infertility (Berg and Denison, 2003).

The following section evaluate the set of aspects which tend to influence the attitude of societies including those of Oman towards practices of female genital mutilation.

### 1.2.1 Influence of culture

An individual acquires most of his social conditions during childhood, before puberty. In childhood, an individual has the capacity to absorb information and follow the examples that exist in his/her social environment, such as the parents and other adults. However, this is constrained by the physical environment: wealth or poverty, threats or security, the level of technology. Furthermore, all human groups, from the nuclear family to the society, develop cultures. (Hofstede, 2003). Hofstede further argues that no group or culture is superior to another: "Cultural Relativism asserts that a culture has no absolute criterion which allows it to judge the activities of another culture as being 'low' or 'noble'." Culture can also be differentiated at national and regional level (given that a large number of countries have very different groups), ethnic, religious, linguistic, gender, generation or social class.

Regarding gender, Hofstede (2003) explains why it is so difficult to change some traditions based on gender:

> If we recognize that within each society there may be a culture that differs from a woman's culture, this helps explain why it is difficult to change traditional gender roles. Feelings and fears about behaviors by the opposite sex can be of the same order of intensity the reactions of people exposed to foreign cultures. The degree of gender differentiation in a country is highly dependent on its national culture.

In terms of equality, a great deal of improvements has been seen in the culture of Oman. According to Al-Hinai (2014), acceptance of women by the society of Oman in an equal manner has come a long way since 1970. Progressive measures have been made to secure the rights of woman in a country that attempts to eliminate the various restrictions that were previously brought down by culture on the women of this country. A new culture of awareness and education has merged as indicated in Oman's Five years plan of Health Ministry for 2006-2010. It was announced that prevalence of FGM/C in Oman will be subjected to research and study for bringing the desired level of awareness among masses (Al-Hinai, 2014).

Jaffer et al(2006) conducted a study to measure the knowledge and beliefs of adolescences in schools revealing shocking insights on the practices of FGM/C. The study revealed that 80% of the girls and boys included in the study showed approval for FGM/C practices. Hence, it is not merely a matter of gender inequality in Oman but of an inclination in the whole culture towards acceptance of these practices. On record, only limited information may be available for the presence of such practices and it may appear that FGM/C is rarely practiced any more, however, the practice may be more common than it has been reported. Abdalla (1982) states that FGM/C is a common practice in Oman among the Omani nationals; Type I which is a partial or total removal of the clitoris and/or the prepuce is commonly practiced in Oman.

## 1.2.2 Influence of tradition

According to the World Health Organization (2001), traditions are a set of customs, beliefs, and values of a community that drive and influence the behavior of its members. They are habits seized, passed from generation to generation and that is part of the identity of a community. Members reproduce these behavioral patterns, believing they are correct and essential, not questioning them in most cases. These traditions are also occasionally protected by taboos, associated with magical and sacred powers, so they are difficult to change. Examples of harmful traditions include, in addition to FGM/C, forced marriage (especially of children with adults), bride buying and early motherhood, food taboos for pregnant women and children, in the search for healthcare decisions made only by men and extended family. Traditions are, in general, linked to shared beliefs, attitudes, and values within a community (a group of people living in the same neighbourhood and sharing an identity, cultural, ethnic and religious characteristics) that pass from generation to generation, until they become an intrinsic part of a culture.

Beliefs can be described as a "conviction", principle or idea accepted as true or real, even without factual evidence. There are numerous "beliefs and belief systems–religious, cultural, group, and individual". Beliefs guide individual actions and behaviors. Values are "moral principles, beliefs or beliefs accepted by an individual or social group. Personal lead people to shape their decisions. Although many values are inherited from families and relatives, they might get influenced by religion, friendships, culture, in addition to educational and personal experiences". Finally, attitudes are "mental approaches or dispositions for something. They are fundamentally based on personal values and perceptions" (WHO, 2001: 65).

Beliefs, attitudes, and values are built and developed under a wide range of influences–family, society, culture, traditions, religion, membership groups, media, climate, technology, politics, economics, experiences, friendships and personal needs by age and gender. A value system is a "hierarchical set of principles that influence the approach (attitude) to the life of a particular person or group, guiding their behavior. As such, it is not rigid but is subject to change over time and according to exposure to new understandings, information and experiences" (WHO, 2001: 65)

Even if the practices of FGM/C are officially banned in the hospitals of Oman, ***the practice has still not been criminalized in the country.*** Similar to its neighbouring Gulf countries, there is little published data that can measure the widespread of FGM/C in Oman. In a report that was published in 2014 after a two weeks field trip in Oman, Wettig points to the fact that

> ***Oman is not on the map of countries where female genital mutilation is practised.*** Neither the United Nations nor international NGOs have taken notice of FGM in the Gulf region – except Yemen. Yet, there are quite a number of reports about its existence in Oman and in most other countries on the Arabian Peninsula, some old from the 1960s, others are medical studies about cysts and other complications.

The deepened roots of the practice in local cultures have posed challenges to the prevention of practices. The situation is more prevalent among conservative communities of Oman where women are seen as symbols of family's honor that can affect the social standing of the whole family. So, it is commonly believed that the sexual desires of young girls must be controlled through such practices. Shawawi Oman mentions on her blog that, traditionally women in Oman have higher beliefs about the practices of FGM/C. According to a study conducted in 2014, seventy-eight percent of the women reported having experienced the process (Human Rights submission, 2017). Majority of these women stated that they were subjected to the process at home due to which no official record could be found of it. Astonishingly, sixty four percent of these women admitted to the fact that the practice of female circumcision was still conducted by their families.

The reason why female circumcision still exist is due to the fact that majority of the population following this in Oman is confused about the religious point of view about the issue. Circumcision is mandated for a male in Islam, however, there is no clear stance given on the practice for women that keeps false beliefs carried in the tradition of the country (Oman and Oman, 2018).

### 1.2.3 Influence of cultural diversity

The United Nations Educational, Scientific and Cultural Organization (UNESCO) is the sole agency of the United Nations in charge of culture. UNESCO recognizes "the equal dignity of all cultures, respect for cultural rights, the formulation of cultural policies for the promotion of diversity, the promotion of constructive pluralism, the preservation of cultural heritage," by way of example. The text of its Constitution (1946) entrusts to it the mission of promoting the diversity of cultures, especially through communication. In the last decades, cultural diversity has been intensifying, due to growing globalization, acquiring "diverse forms through time and space. This diversity manifests itself in the originality and plurality of identities that characterize the groups and societies that make-up humanity. As a source of interchange, innovation, and creativity, cultural diversity is as necessary to mankind as biological diversity to nature. In this sense, it constitutes the common heritage of humanity and must be recognized and consolidated for the benefit of present and future generations" (UNESCO, 2002).

In 2001, UNESCO adopted the Universal Declaration on Cultural Diversity (published in 2002), which argues that "cultural diversity is the heritage of humanity" (Article 1) and is still a development factor and should be preserved (Article 3). However, Article 4, warns that "no one can invoke cultural diversity neither to violate the human rights guaranteed by international law nor to limit their scope". This is the point where the grey area is entered when the problem of FGM/C practices is analysed for Oman (Blanchfield & Browne, 2013).

The UNESCO Convention on the Protection and Promotion of the Diversity of Cultural Expressions (2005) also affirms that this diversity is a fundamental characteristic of humankind, which must be protected and promoted. In addition, the Agenda 2030 for Sustainable Development of the United Nations Organization (2015) includes the role of cultural diversity as an essential element for sustainable development (objective 4, goal 4.7). The diverse cultures of rural and urban areas of Oman create a major barrier towards the understanding and nature of FGM/C practices in the country that is needed to cater the health care problems associated with it. According to Shawawi Oman, the mild form of practice is widely accepted by women across the country for sanitary or religious purposes. (Oman, 2018).

### 1.2.4 Influence of intercultural dialogue

"Intercultural Dialogue is an open, respectful exchange" of ideas based on mutual understanding between "individuals and groups with different ethnic, cultural, religious and linguistic" origins and heritage. Intercultural dialogue is exercised at all levels–within societies, between European societies and between "Europe and the rest of the world" (COE, 2008: 13). According to the White Paper (COE, 2008: 21), it is essential that there are freedom and capacity for expression, as well as the ability to listen to other opinions, so that intercultural dialogue can promote and contribute to "political, social, cultural and economic integration", as well as to the "cohesion of culturally diverse societies". Furthermore, it "fosters equality, human dignity and the feeling of common goals; aims at promoting a better understanding of the diverse practices and visions of the world, strengthening cooperation and participation (or freedom of choice), enabling the development and adaptation of individuals and, finally, promoting tolerance and respect for others". Intercultural dialogue can serve a number of objectives, in the context of the primary objective of promoting respect for human rights and democracy. Jaffer et al(2006) states that an Omani official at the Ministry of Health commented on the data collected from the 2004 survey (Jaffer, Afifi, Al Ajmi & Alouhaishi, 2006) that she was "'unprepared and Shocked' by the unusually high degree of approval, believing until now that the practice was rare and on the decline"("Female Circumcision in Oman", 2005). Intercultural Dialogue is practiced by taking the research and studies on health care concerns associated with FGM/C practices and creating awareness among people of Oman.

## 1.2.5 Influence of discrimination

According to Article 1 of the Convention on the Elimination of all Forms of Discrimination against Women (1979), discrimination against women consists of "Any distinction, exclusion or restriction based on sex and which has the effect or human rights, and fundamental freedoms in the political, economic, social, cultural, and civil" fields, in accordance with the principle of "equality of men and women" or in any other field . Gender inequality continues to be an obstacle to human development, often discriminating against girls and women, preventing access to health, education and political representation (Meyer, 2015).

The Gender Inequality Index, created by the United Nations Development Program (UNDP), measures gender inequalities in three areas of human development: **a)** reproductive health, which is measured by the ratio of maternal mortality and maternal mortality rate; **b)** empowerment, which is measured by the proportion of parliamentary seats held by women and the proportion of adult women and men with some minimum education; and **c)** economic status, which is measured through labor participation among women and men from the age of 15 and onwards. (Assembly, 1979).

Article 17 of the Basic Law of Oman has imposed a prohibition on discriminating practices on the basis of gender. For eliminating all forms of discrimination against women, Oman has subjected Convention on the Elimination of all Forms of Discrimination against Women (CEDAW) to ratifications in 2006. The optional protocol is yet to be ratified (Gender index for Oman, 2018).

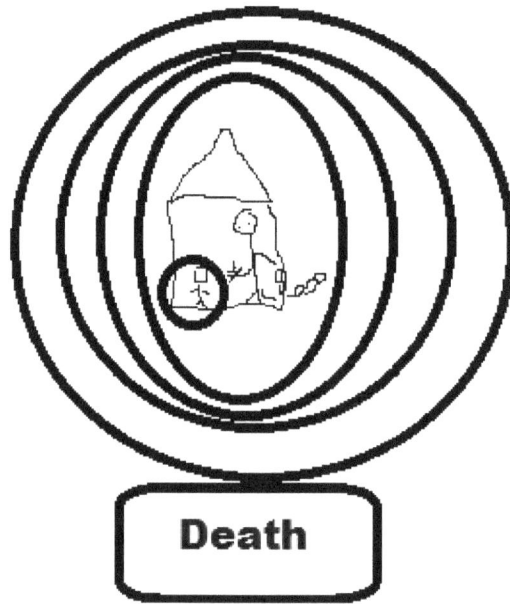

Death

# Chapter Two: Sexual and Reproductive Rights of Women at Local and Global Scales

In addition to violating the rights of children and women, FGM/C also violates the sexual and reproductive rights of these girls and women, as it deprives them of making decisions about their own bodies and hampers access to sexual and reproductive health information, education, and services. In addition to FGM/C, there are other examples of issues related to this type of rights that include (but are not limited to): comprehensive sex education, criminalization and other restrictions on safe abortion, child and forced marriage, violence based in gender, gender equality, gender identity and expression, HIV / AIDS, maternal morbidity and mortality (Chandra-Mouli et al, 2015).

Physical integrity, or the right to the security and control of one's own body, constitutes the core of sexual and reproductive freedom. FGM/C and Human Rights are associated with gender inequality and discrimination and constitute a serious undermining of women's physical and mental health, including their sexual and reproductive lives. Countries are witnessing a human rights violation of countless girls and women whose health and right to life are put at risk. In addition,

35

it may also be linked to other problems such as rape, forced marriages and domestic violence (Gilbert, 2017).

According to WHO (2001), there are several "conventions and declarations that support the promotion and protection of the health of children and women, and some promote the elimination of FGM", such as the aforementioned Declaration of Human Rights (1948). Article 3 stipulates that "everyone has the right to life, liberty and security". The International Covenant on Civil and Political Rights and the International Covenant on Economic, Social and Cultural Rights (1966) condemns gender discrimination, recognizing the universal right of all human beings to the best levels of physical and mental health (Barrett, 2014).

The Convention on the Elimination of all Forms of Discrimination against Women (1979) also calls for the elimination of prejudices and practices that are not based on equality. In addition to the instruments already mentioned, there are still treaties, consensuses and other documents that protect the rights of these girls and women:

**Convention Relating to the Status of Refugees (1967);**

**International Covenant on Civil and Political Rights (1976);**

**International Covenant on Economic, Social and Cultural Rights (1976);**

**Convention on the Elimination of All Forms of Discrimination Against Women (1979);**

**Convention on the Rights of the Child (1990);**

**UN General Assembly Declaration on the Elimination of Violence against Women (1993);**

**Program of Action of the International Conference on Population and Development (1994);**

**Declaration and Platform for Action of the Fourth World Conference on Women in Beijing (1995).**

FGM/C is seen at the international level as a form of gender-based violence and as a harmful tradition that accentuates inequalities and the already unbalanced distribution of power, reducing autonomy and control of women over their own bodies, health, and life, while preventing them from participating equally with men in society. The United Nations Millennium Development Goals (2000-2015) also mention that it is extremely important to promote gender equality and empower women, reduce child mortality, improve maternal health, and combating HIV / AIDS, malaria and other diseases.(Saul et al, 2014; WHO, 2015)

Although the Ministry of Health in Oman acknowledged in its Five- Year Health Plan 2006-2010, that the percentage of circumcised Omani female children (less than 3 years) was 100% in some governorates, which, as it stated "is a matter of concern"("Health Systems Profile- Oman", 2006), until this date, there is no published national data available that would allow for an assessment of the size of the problem in Oman. Kutscher (2011) elaborates that "the silence on the practice might not be so much a sign of the non-incidence of the problem, as of the strength of the taboo imposed on sexuality"

## 2.1 Female Genital Mutilation / Cutting

### 2.1.1 The practice concept

FGM/C as a practice violates a set of fundamental human rights, norms, and principles of gender equality and non-discrimination, as well as the inalienable right "to life and the right to be free from torture", inhumane treatment or degrading (Wadesango et al, 2011). According to the World Health Organization (WHO), it is estimated that more than 200 million girls and women worldwide live with the consequences of FGM/C, and despite efforts to eliminate FGM/C, the 3 million of girls and women are at risk and are therefore exposed to possible negative health consequences (WHO, 2016). The term female genital mutilation, refers to all procedures involving the partial or total removal of the external genitalia or any damage inflicted on the female genitalia for non-medical reasons. FGM/C "violates a number of human rights principles, such as principles of gender equality and non-discrimination, the right to life (when the procedure results in death) and the right not to be subjected to inhuman and degrading punishment, as well as the rights of the child and of the woman"(WHO, 2016). This issue is understood as a clear social problem based on issues of gender discrimination and stigmatization, rooted in asymmetries of power, reflecting one of the many forms of violence against women–physical, psychological, sexual–and with dire consequences for the health, education and empowerment of children, youth and women victims of this practice (Baron and Denmark, 2006).

## 2.1.2 Historical contextualization

Female circumcision already existed in ancient Rome, 5000 years ago (Katania et al, 2007). At the time, in the territory of ancient Egypt there were stratified societies with tight methods of controlling "fidelity", especially in socially high families (Lightfoot-Klein, 1989). Infibulation, still known today as Pharaonic / Sudanese circumcision, was a "form of differentiation between the richer and poorer groups, the symbol of a 'good marriage'" (Mackie, 2000). It can then be concluded that since then, the practice was used as an instrument to control women and their sexuality. However, there are other documents that report that FGM/C began in Egypt and Sudan, and later dispersed due to trade and arranged marriages between Arab nomadic tribes (Oberreiter, 2008). That is, its origin is not consensual.

Cerejo(2017) points to forensic analyses that revealed that the Egyptian mummies showed signs of practice. Other theories also suggest that it has begun with the spread of Islam to some regions of sub-Saharan Africa, and others that may have begun between specific sub-Saharan African ethnic groups and as an integral part of pubertal rites (WHO, 2001: 47). Like Freud's theory (1931), in ancient Egypt it was believed that the clitoris represented the male part of the female (and the foreskin the female part of the male).

Thus, FGM/C and male circumcision were practiced with the aim of differentiating the two genders, so that their responsibilities and roles were clearly separated socially (Martingo, 2009: 47).

In addition, it is believed that this partial removal of the genitals will increase the girls' femininity, that is, it will make them more docile and obedient (Amnesty International, 1997): "It is possible that the trauma of excision may effect on the personality of a girl. If excision is part of a ritual of initiation, then it is accompanied by the teaching on the role of a woman in society" (AI, 1997). It is also believed that Sarah, Abraham's wife, was the first female that carried the practice of circumcision against her Egyptian slave Hagar. Sarah was a sterile woman. Abraham chose Hagar, the Egyptian slave when Sarah suggested to him to take another woman who can give him descendants. However, when Sarah realized Abraham's interest in Hagar, she decided to mutilate Hagar's sexual organ (Robinett, 2006).

Female genital mutilation/cutting, is a very old practice, even before the appearance of monotheistic religions. Neither its origin nor its place of birth is completely clear. Some historians have established that in ancient Egypt the excision was practiced, between 5000 and 6000 BC, during the time of the Pharaohs, hence it is also called "Pharaonic circumcision". One of the reasons that it was practiced was to differentiate the females who came from the upper social class. Some experts have been able to find mutilated sex organs in bodies of mummified women. The specific name of infibulation has its origin during ancient Rome, and comes from the word "fibula", whose name received the brooch with which the Roman women's togas were closed. Closing of the female genital organs was practiced to keep the female virgin before getting married. The reasons were to protect the female from sexual relations with anyone other than her husband, to reduce her sexual desire and to prevent her from being unfaithful to her husband (Martingo, 2009).

During the 17th and 19th centuries female circumcision was practiced in Europe and the United States for supposedly medical reasons. There are also some cases that occurred at the beginning of 20th century. During the 19th century there were some debates in England, on whether circumcision could cure from hysteria, "excessive" masturbation, epilepsy or a migraine. In the case of Africa, FGM/C originates in Egypt and from there it spread to the rest of Africa. Before its colonization, Africa was composed of a large number of ethnic groups that possessed their own autonomy and sovereignty (UNESCO, 2005).

FGM/C, as a practice, accompanies migrant populations, thus becoming a concern of many European countries that welcome these populations who adopt FGM/C as an integral part of a cultural tradition that they carry. At the same time, new population dynamics brought the incidence of FGM/C to countries around the world, where it was traditionally not practiced. Europe, North America, Australia and New Zealand are regions of the globe where the end of FGM/C has become a pressing concern. For example, a report produced for England and Wales states that in these two countries there are only 10,000 girls who have been or will still be subjected to FGM/C. Consistent practice data point to 127,000 women residing in the two countries (Macfarlane & Dorkenoo, 2014). In 2015, Oman Gulf News published about two Omani students who were "studying for their master's degree at UK universities, were arrested and questioned by police in London after approaching a hospital to circumcise their daughters"(Al Mukrashi, 2015).

Migrants carry with them a set of values, beliefs and rituals (cultural) that become part of their trajectories and experiences. This frame of reference that builds the identity of the migrant, particularly when we talk about the phenomenon of FGM/C, intersects with macro-sociological elements such as ethnicity, nationality and gender, and it is crucial to approach practice through the link between them. As Russell points out, "an intersectional approach has been proposed as the only approach one can take to migration to fully represent the complexity of migrants' identities, experiences and trajectories. And yet intersectional analyses often only include gender, nationality, class, "race", and ethnicity, with religion mentioned in passing an attribute of ethnicity" (2012: 760).

These customs have so much weight for the individuals because with them they have the conception that they are part of a community, they are not individual persons, but members of the same community, that without the community they would not exist. And if they do not comply with what their community imposes, they would be attacking the other members of the same community and should be punished, even with death, depending on the crime they have committed. That is why it is so difficult to get them to abide by what is established in the Human Rights Charter and thus avoid the violation of women's rights and mistreat them through traditional practices that are so damaging, since in most cases, the provisions of our regulations fight against the values of their communities (UNESCO,2016). These values of each community are so strong because all the members interrelate with each other. Each member has a specific function, but the gender division is very present.

In the case of women, the functions assigned to them are two: the reproductive function and that of preserving what is produced, that is, feeding and caring for the members of their family. In contrast, the role of men is to work in agriculture, livestock, defending their community, etc. This division of roles is so marked because they live in a patriarchal society in which man protects the community and his family, while women are relegated to the reproductive and domestic sphere. However, the functions exercised by women are vital for the survival of the community and therefore are very controlled by the other members of the same community. ***Moreover, women themselves contribute to violence against girls and other women in their community by engaging in harmful practices, such as using female genital mutilation, or forcing girls and adolescents into forced marriages*** (UNESCO, 2005).

When it does not produce death due to haemorrhage infections -for example, the transmission of HIV or the transmission of hepatitis C caused by the use of the same instrument for multiple operations without proper sterilization-, mutilation of female genitals leaves irreversible such as infertility, lesions of adjacent tissues, kidney injuries, cysts, stones, sexual desire, depression, anxiety, psychosis and serious problems during menstruation, urination, intercourse, pregnancy and childbirth. The fact that sexual mutilations are a traditional practice in some countries from which immigrants originate in the countries of the European Union cannot, in any case, serve as a justification for not preventing, prosecuting and punishing such brutality (Onuh et al, 2016).

## 2.2 FGM / C is a violation of the human rights

FGM/C is acknowledged to be a serious violation of the human rights of females of all ages. We understand the issue as a clear social problem based on gender discrimination and stigmatization, rooted in power asymmetries, reflecting one of the many forms of violence against women–physical, psychological, sexual–and with dire consequences for the health, education and empowerment of children, youth and women victims of this practice. The up-to-date review presented here uses two types of available bibliographic sources. First, on the one hand it reports on: prevalence of FGM/C in countries where it is documented (identified later); prevalence rates in host countries of migrant communities from practicing countries; consequences for the health of women and children; and implementation of public policies to combat FGM/C and the legal framework that punishes and criminalizes this practice (in some countries) as an act of violence against women and children (which prevents them from exercising, among others, the right to identity and full citizenship) (Onuh et al, 2016).

Second, on the other hand, it reports on: academic and scientific studies that focus on the practice and attempt to deconstruct FGM/C from the point of view of perceptions and inculcation of specific cultural beliefs, values, and attitudes in which FGM/C is viewed as a culturally supported practice and identity of some communities and/or countries. With this study, the research team will produce new knowledge in the scientific and academic framework so that the implementation of public policies for the elimination of FGM/C is increasingly effective and sustained. FGM/C, as a practice, "violates a set of fundamental human rights, norms, and principles of gender equality and non-discrimination, as well as the inalienable right to life and the right to be free from torture or cruel" (WHO, 2008).

The Program of Action for the Elimination of Female Genital Mutilation adds that FGM/C "is practiced in some countries of the Arabian Peninsula, such as Oman, Yemen, Bahrain and the United Arab Emirates, as well as in some regions of Indonesia and Malaysia". As Martingo points out, "the term Female Genital Surgery is associated with an implicit acceptance that this practice is performed by health professionals, in a hospital setting. The justification that is often used is that, as it is performed by professionals and with good hygiene and asepsis conditions, it reduces the level of pain and risk (Kaplan et al, 2011). Associated with this designation is thus what is referred to as the medicalization of genital cutting, an issue that has been widely debated in the European context and is the target of the greatest opposition by human rights organizations" (2009: 28).

There are several international organizations that intend to work towards the eradication of FGM/C, both from the point of view of an implementation of public policies, prevention, and sensitization of communities, as well as criminalization and criminalization of the practice. The United Nations began to draw attention to the phenomenon in the late 1970s when FGM/C was still considered only a health issue. The same organisation now regards the phenomenon as something that distorts women and girls in an experience where they are denied the right to equality, health, education, not to be tortured, not to be violated, etc. This resolution reflects international recognition of the seriousness of the phenomenon and the overwhelming need for countries to take action to combat it (EIGE, 2013b). We could not fail to mention the joint declaration of 2008 which brought together 10 United Nations entities and which, based on new evidence and accumulated experience, underlines the fact that the fight against FGM/C requires a coordinated social convention with the various organizations and the communities practicing FGM/C (APF, 2009).

The Council of Europe has also defined policies and recommendations on FGM/C on its agenda. As an example, in 2009, resolution 166215 reaffirms what concrete measures should be taken and that member states should use all the international instruments necessary for the prevention, protection of victims and possible victims and punishment of those responsible. This resolution leads in 2011 to a historic milestone, even by its broader nature in combating gender-based violence and violence against women: the creation of the Council of Europe Convention on the Prevention and Combat of Violence against Women and Domestic Violence (or Istanbul Convention (CoE, 2011)). The importance of this convention lies in the fact that it is "the first legally binding instrument in Europe to prevent and combat violence against women as well as the most far-reaching international treaty to tackle serious violations of women's rights" (EIGE, 2013b: 35). Article 38 of this Convention refers specifically to FGM/C and measures to be taken by Member States: preventive measures, measures to protect victims and concerted efforts to coordinate and understand the phenomenon for the implementation of public policies.

The European Parliament has also been active in producing resolutions aimed at eradicating the phenomenon. In 2001, it adopted the first resolution on FGM/C (European Parliament, 2001), considering the practice as a serious violation of human rights. In 2007, a number of resolutions were adopted with a focus on reproductive health, the status of women from minority groups, development, and violence against women, the rights of the child and FGM/C. The latest resolution on the phenomenon of FGM/C dates from June 2012 and aims at the end of practice, stipulating clearly that "any form of female genital mutilation" is a harmful " practice" (EIGE, 2013b: 38). FGM/C is defined as a practice that affects "the rights and health of women", and in many cases result in the death of these women and girls.(Earp, 2014).

The affects of FGM/C can be serious and persisting during a lifetime. For example FGM/C can cause "genital and urinary infections, pains and lacerations during sexual intercourse, haemorrhages and obstetric fistulas causing pain, disability, infertility"(Gonçalves, 2005: 3). Among the most serious health consequences for women and children, the EIGE report (2013b) states that the risk of contracting HIV and other sexually transmitted infections is greater. In addition to the above consequences, girls or women may exhibit some of the following symptoms: difficulty draining secretions and menstrual blood, recurrent urinary infection, scarring fibrosis. As for obstetric complications, consequences such as obstruction of labor, rupture of the tissues, prolongation of the expulsive period, can also result from an increase in the number of cesarean sections, fetal distress and prolonged and painful labor (Campos, 2010). ). Other health professionals report that the occurrence of "sebaceous or inclusion cysts (dermoid cysts), keloid, ulcer, neurinoma, and dysmenorrhea" may also be recorded (Vicente, 2007: 91). The experience of women's sexuality is equally affected. The decrease and/or absence of sensitivity and sexual pleasure, dyspareunia, difficulty in vaginal penetration and anorgasmia, with the consequences of the psychological forum are revealed in the fear of the occurrence of sexual relations and in many cases are manifested through post-traumatic stress disorder (Vicente, 2007). In this sense, the experience of the sexuality of the women or girls subjected to the practice is affected. For example, vaginal penetration through injured and scarred genital tissue may be difficult or impossible, with rupture of the tissue, causing further bleeding and severe pain(Onuh,2006). Until this date the research on the psychological consequences of FGM/C remains limited. However, few studies reflect an increased "fear of sexual intercourse, post-traumatic stress disorder, anxiety, depression and memory loss". (Berg and Danisson, 2015).

## 2.2.1 The support for mutilation is declining

The practice of genital ablation is concentrated in localized areas of Africa, the Middle East, Asia and Latin America, a list that includes 29 countries. However, in most of these places, there is a marked social rejection of this practice, as documented by the United Nations Children's Fund (UNICEF). Over the years, support for mutilation has declined, even in countries where it was entrenched, such as Egypt. According to the latest data from the agency, if the countries where it is still practiced are taken into account globally, 67% of women and 63% of men think that it should be eliminated. "In some countries such as Senegal, Cameroon or Cote d'Ivoire, this rejection exceeds 80%". (UNICEF, 2016) However, the studies on perceptions of women in Oman have indicated different results. In a paper, titled *Towards a solution concerning female genital mutilation?*, Kutscher (2011) argues that "this does not imply that the practice is non-existent in these places. In fact, the Arabian Peninsula is frequently named among the regions where FGM is or was common". In its 2014 analysis about Oman, UN WOMEN reported that "female genital mutilation (FGM) is not a common practice" in the country ("Oman", 2014). However,

According to a 2001 Ministry of Health survey of over 3,500 16-18 year-old, almost 80% of those polled believe that female genital mutilation (FGM) is "necessary and important," with 46.3% of males and 45.1% of females strongly agreeing with the practice. ("Female Genital Mutilation Part of National Action Plan", 2006)

Moreover, another survey was generated in 2004. The statistics

revealed that 85% of females of all ages accept FGM as a practice, with 53% having had the procedure done themselves (46% had partial cutting, 8% had the most severe form of FGM, and 46% had no form of FGM). ("Female Genital Mutilation Part of National Action Plan", 2006)

## 2.3 Is FGM/C a cultural or a religious tradition?

Female genital mutilation is considered an extreme manifestation of sexist violence against women because it is so and is linked to other abuses, such as forced marriage. Its origins are not clear, but, according to the United Nations Population Fund (UNFPA), they pre-date the beginnings of Islam and Christianity. "No religion promotes this practice", insist on the specialized agency. The ablation is practiced by some Muslim groups, by certain Christian and Jewish groups, as well as by the followers of some animistic religions. It is a cultural tradition, not religious, that responds to several reasons. First, as UNICEF summarizes, it seeks to diminish sexual desire in women, maintains their virginity before marriage and fidelity. Second, it means "the initiation of girls into adulthood". The impoverishment of women in societies where ablation is a prerequisite to marriage also influences. Some communities consider, on the other hand, that the female genitalia is "little clean and unsightly" with respect to deeply rooted ideals of beauty and purity. Ultimately, it is sometimes practiced "under the mistaken belief" that some religions demand it. According to the UNFPA, the more widespread the practice, the more condemnation, harassment, and uprooting can be suffered by those who decide to deviate from the norm. For this reason, the support of the rest of the community becomes vital so that families can abandon it. Also, there are voices that point to the lack of training of professionals who are in contact with possible victims in Europe, which can lead to the stigmatization of victims (OHCHR,2008).

### 2.3.1 Beliefs and justifications

This millenarian practice happens for several reasons, and these justifications change from country to country, sometimes even from village to village. There are numerous reasons for the continuation of this practice: socio-cultural, economic, psychological, hygienic and aesthetic, spiritual and religious justifications, and even psychosexual justifications. In addition, it is founded on traditional beliefs, values and attitudes. Depending on the country, culture or region, it is believed that this practice increases fertility and facilitates childbirth, improves the level of hygiene and makes the female genitals more beautiful. It is believed that this practice releases a female from a dangerous organ. Moreover, in some cultures, it is believed that the clitoris will render men sterile if their genitals come into contact, or it will kill the newborn. (Behrendt, 2011: 23).

One of the beliefs is that clitoris is a male part; so they are cutting the male part of the female body in order to stop this part from growing ( Behrendt, 2005). In addition, many communities associate FGM/C with supernatural powers, demons and black magic. It is customary to blame these evil spirits when infections occur or even death. "In any society, social inclusion, the feeling of being part of the group, of being accepted by the peers is fundamental to the balance of each element and of the community as a whole" (Marcelino, in APF, 2008: 117). In other communities, it is seen as a way of preserving girls' virginity until marriage (as in Sudan, Egypt, Ethiopia and Somalia): "In every community where FGM is practiced, this is the important part of identity culturally defined gender, which explains why so many mothers and grandparents support the practice: they consider it to be a fundamental part of their femininity and believe it to be essential for the integration of their daughters into society. In most of these communities, FGM/C is a prerequisite for marriage and marriage is vital to women's social survival and economics" (WHO, 2001: 71).

It is important to remember that this procedure is performed by an older woman (Martingo, 2009: 113). For these women, who often also prepare for childbirth, marriage and postpartum procedure, the practice of FGM/C represents a source of economic income for themselves and their families (Alice, 2001). For example, Marzouka who is an Omani traditional cutter from Salalah "cuts two to seven girls a day, she says, making 15 riyals (30 Euros) each" ("Meeting a Circumciser: "Men suffer from it" – In Salalah facing up against FGM is almost impossible", 2013).

For these reasons, it is necessary to realize that these communities have reasons to value FGM/C and that changing traditional values and attitudes is a long process. Only then can they reflect on the practice and see if it results from a rational choice or an influence. For example, in Salalah-Oman, "the idea to not mutilate a girl is unheard of" ("Meeting a Circumciser: "Men suffer from it" – In Salalah facing up against FGM is almost impossible", 2013). According to the United to END FGM (UEFGM) e-learning course of the Mediterranean Institute of Gender Studies, this is a tradition that aims to control female sexuality, since a woman's virginity is seen as a prerequisite for marrying , and is also linked to the honor of the family(Middelburg and Balta,2016). Thus, infibulations is used to reduce female sexual desire (as well as premarital sexual intercourse), preserving and testing female virginity. The course adds that, given that in some societies non-excised women cannot touch water or food, we can also talk about hygiene as a justification used by some cultures: they believe that the female genitalia are something dirty and, therefore, something to eliminate. Also cultural identity is a key factor in this tradition, since it defines who belongs to the community (Bansal et al, 2013).

For example, if in a community this practice is seen as a ritual of initiation, a non-excised girl will not be considered an adult. It also marks the difference between the sexes in terms of their role in marriage and life. "It is understood as a duty of a mother in the preparation of her daughters for her duties as future wives." (Toubia,1995). Although many believe that this is a religious obligation, Behrendt states that this is a cultural practice that precedes Christianity or Islam.(2011: 23). In addition to the above-mentioned consequences, according to the Manfred Nowak report (2008), FGM/C

[I]nvolves the deliberate infliction of severe pain and suffering. The pain is usually exacerbated by the fact that the procedure is carried out with rudimentary tools and without anesthetic. Many girls enter a state of shock induced by the extreme pain, psychological trauma and exhaustion from screaming. The procedure can result in death through severe bleeding leading to haemorrhagic shock, neurogenic shock as a result of pain and trauma, and overwhelming infection and septicaemia. Other immediate medical complications include ulceration of the genital region, injury to adjacent tissues and urine retention.

Nowak(2012) adds that pain caused by FGM/C is not limited to the initial procedure, but generally continues throughout life: "depending on the type and severity of the procedure", there might be long-term health problems such as "chronic infections, tumors , abscesses, cysts, infertility, excessive growth of scar tissue, increased risk of HIV / AIDS infection, hepatitis". Also, FGM/C might damage the urethra which can result in urinary incontinence and painful menstruations. FGM/C also increases the risk of death of the mother and child during childbirth, and even higher incidences of postpartum hemorrhages.

Nowak (2008) further writes that women who are infibulated must be dis-infibulated later, such as during marriage and during childbirth, causing even more physical and psychological problems. This happens through surgery or even during sexual intercourse, which increases pain during the first few weeks, in addition to the pain and complications that man can experience.

WHO (2014) has estimated that "100 to 140 million girls and women have already been subjected to one of the forms of Female Genital Mutilation / Cutting and that at least 3 million are at risk annually, or 8000 per day". Most of them originate in 29 African countries (Benin, Burkina Faso, Cameroon, Chad, Congo, Côte d'Ivoire, Djibouti, Egypt, Eritrea, Ethiopia, Gambia, Ghana, Guinea, Guinea Bissau, Liberia, Mali, Mauritania Senegal, Sierra Leone, Somalia, Sudan, Tanzania, Togo and Uganda). There are also some countries and regions in the Middle East (Saudi Arabia, Yemen, Iraq and some Kurdish communities), in Asia (Indonesia) and in "some ethnic groups in Central and South America that maintain this tradition, such as the Embera people in Colombia, where FGM/C is performed on newborns". It was introduced in this community in the eighteenth century, through the presence of African slaves from Mali (Cosoy, 2016).

WHO (2014) further notes that FGM/C is also registered in Israel, Oman and the United Arab Emirates in the Middle East, as well as in India, Sri Lanka and Malaysia in Asia. Type and reasons and a number of girls and women submitted vary from country to country, and even from community to community (UNICEF: 2016). In addition, it is important to note that women undergoing FGM/C are now scattered around the world, largely due to forced migration, as a consequence of globalization.

It is important to realize that, despite having already been banned in many countries, the practice persists, mainly due to reasons associated with culture and tradition, such as: belief that it is a requirement of religion; preservation of virginity / chastity; control of women's sexuality; social acceptance; marriage requirement; ritual of passage; preservation of family honor; gender identity; sense of belonging and identity to a particular group. The anti-FGM/C campaign advocates women's sexual and reproductive rights–a position supported by international human rights law and international law in many European Union countries. The legal precepts regarding the fundamental rights "must be interpreted and integrated in accordance with the Universal Declaration of Human Rights" (Wangila,2015). However, as has already been mentioned, there are no religious foundations that oblige the practice of FGM/C in any of the sacred books: the Old Testament, the Bible and the Quran (Branco, 2006: 59).

The type of mutilation and the age at which girls are excised depends on a number of factors, such as nationality, ethnic group, socioeconomic status of the family and the area: rural or urban. It is usually practiced in children between 4 and 12 years. However, in some cultures the procedure happens at birth, before marriage, or during the first pregnancy, and is usually celebrated by the family and community, marking the transition to adulthood. For example, in "Dhofar, the Southern province of Oman, girls are traditionally mutilated in the first two days of their lives" ("Meeting a Circumciser: "Men suffer from it" – In Salalah facing up against FGM is almost impossible", 2013).In addition, it is important to note that some women are excised more than once during their lifetime, such as after childbirth (very common in infibulation communities), which is called "reinfibulation" (UNICEF, 2005). Human Rights Watch reveals in its study on FGM/C in Yemen, that when a girl was born at a hospital in Oman, it was a "normal procedure for nurses to ask mothers if they wish their girl to be mutilated and then, if mothers agree, it is carried out at the same day of delivery or a day after" (Wille, 2014).

### 2.3.2 The harmful consequences of FGM/C

WHO identifies four types of FGM / C, depending on the greater or lesser extent of this practice (Hicks, 2018). The phrase, female genital mutilation/cutting, FGM/C, gained increasing support in the late 70s. The phrase mutilation establishes a clear linguistic distinction with male circumcision. Also, given its clearly negative connotations, it underlines the seriousness of the act. In

1990, this term was adapted at the Third Conference of the Inter-African Committee on Traditional Practices Affecting the Health of Women and Children, held in Addis Ababa (Johnsdotter, 2009).

World Health Organization estimates that there are 92 million women and girls over 10 years old who have suffered from FGM/C. For example, in Spain there are 10,000 girls who are at risk of suffering ablation. Ablation involves the partial or total mutilation of the external female genitalia of girls and is commonly practiced in the eastern, western, and north-eastern regions of Africa, as well as in some countries in Asia and the Middle East. It is a practice rooted in the societies of these countries that have cultural, social and religious origins (Kaplan, Hechavarría, Martín &Bonhoure, 2011).

Contrary to the popular beliefs of these regions, female genital mutilation without clinical reasons does not entail any health benefit. Immediately, the symptoms that women or girls suffer are intense pain, haemorrhage, tetanus, sepsis, and urinary retention, open sores in the area or injuries to neighbouring genital tissues. All this, without forgetting the fatal immediate consequence: the death of the girl due to exsanguination or due to neurogenic collapse due to the trauma and intense pain. But that is not all, many of them are condemned to suffer in their health the consequences of this practice throughout their lives (Kaplan, Hechavarría, Martín & Bonhoure, 2011).

The practice of FGM/C varies a lot from one country to another. In general, it is usually done on girls from 4 to 12 years old, but in some cultures it is practiced a couple of days after birth, and in others, before marriage or after the first pregnancy. However, according to UNICEF, the average age at which girls are subjected to FGM / C is falling in some countries. It is attributed to a possible consequence of the adoption of national legislation that prohibits it, which has encouraged families to carry out their practice at an earlier age, so that it is easier to hide it before the authorities. It includes "a wide variety of practices that suppose the total or partial extirpation of the external genitalia or its alteration for reasons that are not of a medical nature". This procedure may involve the use of non-sterilized, improvised or rudimentary tools.

In 1991 the World Health Organization (WHO) recommended the United Nations (UN) to adopt this terminology and since then it has been widely used in its documents. In 1999, the UN Special Rapporteur on Traditional Practices called for tact and patience in relation to activities in this particular area and called attention to the risk of "demonizing" certain cultures, religions and communities. As a result, the Ablation term is used more and more to avoid the alienation of certain communities (UNICEF, 2002).

The justifications suggested for its practice are numerous, and in their specific, convincing contexts. Although these justifications may vary between communities, they have a number of common themes: it assures the girl or woman a status, the possibility of getting married, chastity, health, beauty and honors her family. In some cases it is presented as a positive convention when highlighting the advantages of submitting to it, while in others it focuses on the consequences of not submitting to its practice. Among the Chagga of Arusha in Tanzania, the relationship between FGM / C and the value of girls is evident; the price of the bride is much higher in the case that the girl has been subjected to it (Skaine, 2005).

It is also practiced alleging that it preserves the virginity of the girl, which makes the intervention a prerequisite for marriage. In Nigeria, for example, "it has the purpose of allowing the future mother-in-law to verify the virginity of the bride". Equally, it is often justified that it protects females from experiencing too many sexual desires and accordingly "helps preserve their morality, chastity and fidelity". In addition, it can be associated with body hygiene and beauty.

For example, in Somalia and Sudan, infibulation is practiced for the purpose of females being physically clean. There are also religious reasons that defend the practice. In numerous cases, those communities that cite a religious reason consider FGM/C a requirement for the female to be spiritually pure.

Although there is a theological branch of Islam that supports it, the Sunna type, the Quran does not include any text that requires the ablation of the external genital organs of women and the idea that the practice was among the Sudanese populations and Nubians before the appearance of Islam is widespread (Dorkenoo & Elworthy, 1992). Ablation does not depend on religion and is carried out by both Muslim and Christian or animist communities. In 2010, 34 Muslim scholars of Mauritania dictated a fatwa forbidding genital mutilation (Berg & Denison, 2013). Whether "religious, aesthetic, hygienic or moral, the justifications given are mechanisms" to "maintain the social convention" of subjecting females to this custom and contributing to its perpetuation, information about these justifications "helps to change attitudes towards FGM/C". However, the change in real and definitive attitude is most probably to result from the transformation of the social convention itself.

Female genital mutilation, which consists in the

total or partial amputation of the clitoris and other procedures that injure the female genital organs, is still practiced on girls in some 29 countries (in addition to those that have been the result of emigration), of which 27 are African and affects about 200 million women worldwide. Like the Gambia, Nigeria voted a regulation in 2015 against this ancestral practice, while the African Union Parliament approved a plan of action to eradicate it from the continent, already banned in a total of 23 countries. However, in most of these countries it is still practiced. In countries such as Egypt, Somalia, Guinea or Sudan the rate of mutilated women exceeds 90%. As for Oman, although the practice of FGM/C was banned in the state's health sectors through issuing " a ministerial decree effective from 9th January 2001 prohibiting the practice in government and private health facilities", the government has not introduced any official legislation to ban FGM/C officially. Prior to this ban, FGM/C was "performed openly in Oman with medical supervision in hospitals by trained male and female health professionals" ("Oman", 2013). Until this date, no detailed study has been published by the Omani government on FGM/C in Oman and its strategic plan to address this issue (Ghimire, 2016).

Although the impact on health depends on a set of factors, scope and type of ablation, ability of the person who performs it, type of tool (knife, sharp stone, piece of glass), cleaning tools and environment, and physical state of the woman or girl, FGM/C causes irreversible damage and endangers the health, and even the life, of the affected female. In fact, the most common immediate consequences are intense pain, since it is usually practiced without anesthesia or with local medicines such as herbs. In the medium and long term, the female may suffer superficial infections of the wound due to the use of non-sterilized or contaminated instruments (Berg & Denison, 2013).

Mutilated females can also suffer from various kidney disorders, such as urinary retention (caused by pain, inflammation and infection), or in the case of infibulation, difficulty urinating (the bladder of an infibulated female can take up to 15 minutes to empty), and menstrual disorders (menstruation can be more painful and last longer). In addition, the mutilated female can suffer obstetric complications (longer births, major bleeding, more complications, and the likelihood of needing a c-session since scarring usually hinders the baby's exit through the vaginal canal, and therefore, the child is more likely to die in the perinatal period), and various gynecological problems (infections of the vaginal tract due to obstruction of menstrual flow, infections in the pelvis, cysts, fistulas), and even infertility. On the other hand, the physical damages associated with the trauma can hinder the enjoyment of a normal sexual life, by provoking coital pain, anorgasmia or frigidity, as well as a limitation of sexual pleasure (Committee on Bioethics, 1998; Hicks, 2018).

Regarding the psychological effects, blood loss, pain and fear can generate important traumas during the act and reach the state of medical shock, or later cause psychological and psychosomatic disorders, such as anguish and alterations in eating habits. In addition, a specific syndrome has been identified: genitally focused anxiety-depression, characterized by a constant concern about the state of the genitals and the panic of infertility (Abdulcadir, Rodriguez & Say, 2015). Thus, genital mutilation has harmful consequences for the health of the female, both physical, mental and sexual .

## 2.4 Factors that affect the practice of FGM/C

These factors will serve us to make a spatial, educational, economic and social delimitation, which allows us to better understand the characteristics of the communities that carry out these practices, as well as their members. In addition, it will also help us to better understand the foundations that lead these groups to think and consider what the arguments are for those who perform FGM/C in Oman since for them, this defence is the epicentre of the values of their entire culture (Boyle, 2005). The factors that affect the FGM/C are investigated in the following sections:

## 2.4.1 Education

It has been shown that the higher the educational level of women within a community, the lower the risk of exposing their daughters to female genital mutilation. For this reason, this type of practice is usually associated with communities to which education has not reached the desired level, therefore they are illiterate communities. It is significant that in some countries in which the prevalence of these practices continues to be very high, we can observe how lacking an adequate educational level and therefore not having obtained all the information necessary to prevent them from practising FGM/C on their daughters, they decide to cut their daughters (Hunter collage, 2015). However, it should be noted that this does not occur in all the countries that are shown below, rather it occurs in some cities or towns where it has been impossible to integrate this type of education.

## 2.4.2 Place of residence

It has been shown that the population living in rural areas has higher prevalence rates of FGM/C than populations living in urban areas. For this reason, the migrations from rural areas to urban areas, is helping women who live in villages and who have suffered FGM/C, to receive sufficient information to prevent their daughters from being mutilated genitally, so that the FGM/C rate in urban environments is declining noticeably. In any case, it cannot be generalized, since there are countries such as Nigeria, in which the rate of mothers who mutilate their daughters is high in both rural and urban areas, but in most cases is as we have explained thanks to the migratory processes towards urban areas(GSN, 2006; UNICEF, 2005).

The data referred to African women who have been subjected to FGM/C in rural areas have higher percentages in Mali with 83%, compared to 55% in urban areas; Sudan with 82% in rural areas, compared to 72% in cities; Egypt with 82%, like Sudan in rural areas, and 72% in urban areas; followed by Guinea with 75% compared to 55 in the cities. These countries, being countries with a very high prevalence rate, do not perceive too much the differences between the rural environment and the cities, and this because these practices are deeply rooted throughout the country. On the other hand, it is significant that only Yemen and Nigeria have a higher rate of female genital mutilation in urban areas than in rural areas. Yemen is 22% in the urban environment compared to 20% in rural areas, as we can see that there is hardly any difference between the two areas; while Nigeria does notice this difference, since in urban areas it has a rate of 16% and in rural areas it is 9% (GSN, 2006; UNICEF, 2005).

### 2.4.3 Religion

A single religion cannot be pointed out, as in this case with Islam, to explain why female genital mutilation is performed. However, these statistics are insightful for the case of Oman. The countries, whose majority religion is Muslim, which have rates of genitally mutilated women are: first Mali, with 81% of women professing the Muslim religion compared to 61% of Christian women; second, Sudan, with 79% of Muslim women victims versus 42% of Christian women; Third, we find Ethiopia, with a Muslim female rate of 76% compared to 58% among Christian women; and, fourth, we find Eritrea, which has a prevalence of 73% for victims of these practices who profess the Muslim religion, compared to 32% of Christian women. Be that as it may, it seems striking to note that there are two countries that, although they have a very low rate of mutilation, are more practiced in Christian than Muslim women. These countries are: first, Kenya, with 26% of Christian women, compared to 15% of Muslim women, and second, Nigeria, with 16% of Christian women versus 7% of Muslim women. Although the statistical data show that there is a substantial differentiation between women victims of Muslim and Christian genital mutilation, this data has helped us to eradicate the myth that the practice of FGM/C is a question of

Islam, that is uncertain because, as we have been able to verify, these practices have been carried out long before Islam was established as a religion(GSN, 2006; UNICEF, 2005).

### 2.4.4 Age

Age, without a doubt, is a determining factor, because the education that is being offered to adult women and young women who have not yet had any children is showing positive results, since it is being demonstrated that the levels of FGM/C have descended in young groups aged between 15-19 and 20-24 years. The age groups, whose prevalence in the countries where FGM/C is practiced, are progressively decreasing from 52% in the age group of 45-49 to 38% in the age group of 15 to 19 years. In eastern and southern Africa it is shown how the percentage is decreasing from 52% in the age group of 45 to 49 years, up to 34% in the age group between 15 and 19 years. In contrast, the prevalence in the Middle East and North Africa has declined very little, with the data being as follows: first of all, there is a total of 86% of the female population genitally mutilated in the age group between 45 and 49 years, followed with 85% of the age groups between 40 and 34 years, to finish in 80% in the age group between 15 and 19 years(GSN, 2006; UNICEF, 2005).

Then it can be said that the measures adopted are not

unified, but that each country complies with them in the way it thinks it is necessary, although in many cases the main problem is that the governments of some of them are not aware of the effects produced by this type of practices.

Finally, the decision of mothers to mutilate their daughters depends on several factors related to their own personal experience. In the first place, it depends on the age at which she was genitally mutilated, since if she was not aware of the process she will not stand against the traditions of her community. It also depends on whether the mother has a support group who can protect her if she does not subject her daughter to genital mutilation. (GSN, 2006; UNICEF, 2005). In her 2016 clinical research findings of a study which was conducted at the University College London Hospital on children with FGM, Creighton S. et al reveals that she examined a child who "was allegedly subjected to FGM while on a family holiday in Oman and DVD review confirmed as small scar consistent with type 4 FGM" (Creighton, Dear, de Campos, Williams & Hodes, 2015).

## 2.4.5 Wealth

In its 2005 *Statistical Exploration* on FGM/C, UNICEF shows that "in households whose wealth level is higher, the FGM/C index is lower than in poor households". The analysis of this type is carried out from income quantiles, which consists in dividing the population into five parts or quantiles, from the poorest to the richest. In the case of Africa, within these quantiles are included the properties of the home, such as a television, a car, etc., and are attached to the rest of the dwelling's facilities, as well as the sanitation thereof, etc., and in all of it, individuals are framed by the characteristics of all the properties they possess. For this reason, in countries such as Chad, Benin, Kenya and Mauritania it was found that in 60% of the households where FGM/C had been practiced on women in the family, they were poor households (UNICEF, 2005).

# Chapter Three : Foundations for Establishing and Consolidating FGM/C

### 3.1 Types of female mutilation

According to the World Health Organization (WHO), there are four main types. The first, called clitoridectomy, consists of partial or total resection of the clitoris and, in very rare cases, only of the foreskin. The second is excision and involves, in addition to the clitoris, the resection of the labia minora. Infibulation consists of narrowing of the vaginal opening and repositioning of minor or major lips (with or without clitoral resection). Finally, within the fourth group, a wide range of practices are included, such as perforation, incision, scraping or cauterization of genitals (Mitike & Deressa, 2009).

Often, the ablation is reduced to a single form, the third type, that is, the removal of the labia minora and major and the clitoris, and the subsequent closure of the vagina by suturing. There are, however, three more types, according to the World Health Organization (WHO): the partial or total amputation of the clitoris, the removal of the clitoris and labia minor and, finally, the rest of harmful techniques such as perforation, incision or scraping of the genital area. The effects on the body and the mental well-being of women and girls are many. It can initially produce intense pain, severe (in many cases fatal) haemorrhages and urinary problems. Later it can cause cysts, infections, infertility, and complications of childbirth and increased risk of death of the newborn. In the long term, it can lead to mental health problems such as depression, anxiety and low self-esteem (UNICEF, 2005).

## 3.2 The structure of FGM/C foundations

The foundations for establishing and consolidating FGM/C cover topics of different kinds. They range from cultural traditions, through religion, to aesthetic or hygienic causes. In order to do so, each one of these foundations must be studied in depth, in order to understand what it is that moves the communities to carry out these practices without thinking about the detriment of their realization.

### 3.2.1 Cultural identity

The cultural identity is made up of the knowledge learned by the customs and traditions of the community to which the female belongs. Therefore, cultural identity is perhaps the foundation that most characterizes FGM/C. Since many studies explain that females who undergo these mutilations become members of the group. Moreover, Females who do not undergo this process are defined as "marginalized" or "foreign".

Therefore, in those communities the habit of practicing FGM/C to females is very normal, because otherwise these females would never become adults and could not receive acceptance to live within the borders of the community (Whitehorn et al, 2002; M'jamtu-Sie,2007).

### 3.2.2 Sexual identity

The acquisition of this identity is linked to the cultural identity. In many communities its is believed that the female genital organs, being bulky, are male parts in the woman's body. Therefore the female must go under FGM/C practice to remove the male parts from her body. Only through this practice she is granted to gain femininity. (Alavi, 2003). In addition, initiation rites are accompanied by specific teachings on the role that a female should play within the borders of her community, for example, how to behave with her husband, how to care for her children and how to fulfil her duties towards the members of her community (Sajó, 2013).

### 3.2.3 Control of women's sexuality

In most of the communities where FGM/C is carried out, it is believed that this practice considerably reduces female's sexual desire, and therefore, the husband should not worry that his wife is unfaithful. These practices are carried out because men do not believe that women will be faithful to them voluntarily. In the cases of infibulations, these foundations go further, since they sew and dislodge the woman depending on the sexual need of the husband. For this reason, the communities that mostly practice infibulations are societies where patriarchy is deeply rooted (Glasier et al, 2006).

In some communities, it is believed that having sex with a woman who has not been subjected to genital mutilation can be very dangerous for the man, because the clitoris could cause the death of the man if it has contact with his penis. On the other hand, it is believed that genital mutilation facilitates childbirth because the child shall die instantly if the child rubs the clitoris of the mother at the time of delivery (Sajo, 2013).

### 3.2.4 Hygiene and aesthetics

Cleaning and hygiene are two factors that are systematically shown when referring to female genital mutilation as a ritual of purification. In some communities, women who have not suffered genital mutilation are considered dirty women and are forbidden from handling food or water. Another reason why the female genital organs are removed, is that they are considered ugly and bulky. By cutting the clitoris, the female gains femininity(Earp, 2014).

### 3.2.5 Religion and mythology

There is no direct relationship between religion and FGM/C, but with the passage of time has been acquiring a greater role. In fact, females who refuse to undergo genital mutilation are rejected by the community, and cannot, among other things, go to pray. But these precepts are not exposed either in the Quran or in any other religious manuscript. This problem has persisted throughout history and many missionaries have tried to stop it, but its rootedness is so great that they have had to desist, and even in some cases, approve it. In the case of mythology, there are many myths that refer to the origin of FGM/C. For example in Bambara, which is a village in Mali, it is believed that an evil spirit is lodged in the clitoris, and only through cutting the clitoris this spirit disappears, then the female can purify herself (Momoh, 2017).

### 3.2.6 Sociocultural

In most of the occasions, the social and cultural context in which this practice is framed is the passage of girls to puberty. According to Van Gennep, these rights do not correspond to the onset of physical puberty, since no physiological change is observed, so it is a social puberty, in which the age of initiation varies depending on the ethnicity, the location of the country and population density. The meaning of these rites is of an extraordinary complexity, due to the differences between the tribes that realize it, the country in which it is carried out and the traditions of each group (Van Gennep, 1960). The duration of the healing of the wound depends on the type of FGM/C that has been practiced. (Marcusán, n.d). In addition to being recognized as adults, mutilated females are also accepted, legitimized and assigned the role they will follow for the rest of their lives (Xiong, n.d).

Female genital mutilation is practiced in 29 African and Asian countries. However, its effects are seen in many countries where these families migrate. It is estimated that some 140 million women and girls suffer from problems due to this technique or the conditions under which it is performed (UNICEF, 2005). They range from intense pain to haemorrhages or infections (instruments such as knives, glasses, cans ... that are not sterilized are used). There are also lesions of organs and anatomical structures of the area (urethra, vagina, perineum or rectum). Due to malpractice, infections such as HIV, hepatitis or tetanus can be acquired. Menstrual pains are greater as are genitourinary fistulas, incontinence, cysts or retention of menstrual content in the vagina (Nour, 2008).

### 3.3 Legal framework for Oman

Due to numerous campaigns to raise awareness of FGM/C, which are organised by the local and global organizations that fight for the human rights of women and children , many countries in which FGM/C was considered a legalized practice, decided to prohibit the FGM/C practice and to issue sanctioning laws. Moreover, to classify FGM/C as a crime, several states in Europe, such as Norway, Sweden, United Kingdom, have passed specific laws and several states have modified their legislation, such as Austria, Belgium, Denmark and Spain. In many European states, for example, Germany, Finland, France, Greece, Italy, the Netherlands and Switzerland, among others, FGM/C is legally forbidden under the application of general criminal laws and is usually assimilated to an attack against the physical and moral integrity of the person.

In recent years new studies are showing that FGM/C is also practiced in the Middle East. Among the Middle Eastern countries are those that are known as the Gulf countries such as Oman, Bahrain,Qatar, Kuwait and United Arab Emirates(Geraci & Mulders, 2016) . However, because "no nationally representative data exist" UNICEF reveals that its "understanding remains limited" generally on FGM/C prevalence in the Middle East and particularly in this region of Gulf countries, for example Oman. ("Leveraging Education to End Female Genital Mutilation/Cutting Worldwide", 2016)

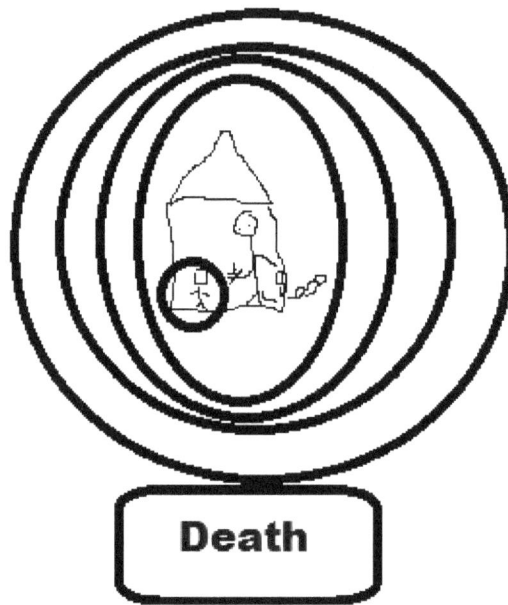

Death

# Chapter Four : Conclusion

The fact that female genital mutilation is exercised against women because they are female leads researchers to describe ablation as another form of sexist violence. However, until recently it was not considered as such because it was justified through cultural practices, and the female victims are considered inferior and owned by men, remaining in oblivion and giving impunity to the perpetrators. In addition, we must not forget that, when occurring in the home, was considered a space outside the control of the states, a private matter of families, closing their eyes to this reality. It has not been until recently when the United Nations has qualified it as a violation of the Human Rights of women and girls, and it was the WHO in the 70s who put the spotlight on it. However, it is not until 1993 within the framework of the Declaration on the Elimination of Violence against Women, when it is recognized that cultural traditions and customs should not serve to undermine the integrity of girls and women, and that those practices that they do so must be eliminated. Consequently, female genital mutilation is prohibited in most of the countries where it is practiced, but it does not prevent it from being practiced. Of 29 countries where it is practiced, ablation is prohibited in 25, but the law is practically powerless.

## 4.1 Short term and long term consequences reported in literature

Among the main dangers and consequences for health that genital mutilation entails are severe pain, bleeding, difficulty urinating and even defecation, the possibility of suffering infections due to the use of contaminated instruments. As women who practice mutilation do not understand medicine, they simply cut; girls bleed to death. If they do not die from the pain, they can die from the infection. In addition, according to UN data, girls who suffer this violence are more likely to be infected with AIDS, suffer psychological consequences, imbalances in menstruation, and infections in the urinary system, and complications in childbirth and problems in their quality of sexual life. There is no doubt, therefore, that we are talking about a human rights issue, an attack against the physical integrity of women, and a violation of their sexual and reproductive rights whose consequences harm and mark the bodies and lives of women (Reisel et al, 2015).

FGM/C has both short and long-term consequences on the physical and psychological health of women, since generally the conditions in which they are practiced are neither of maximum asepsis nor the materials are sterilized. FGM/C involves the removal of the clitoris and all of the major and minor lips, leaving a small hole for urine and menstruation. Generally, complications can be distinguished between early or late (Berg and Underland, 2013).

### 4.1.1 Early

The bulbar area usually has abundant irrigation and innervations, which causes intense pain associated with fear and anguish that can cause a neurogenic shock. Pain hinders urination that causes urinary retention. Bleeding, if not controlled, can cause hypovolemic shock and cause death (Berg and Danison, 2012).

### 4.1.2 Delays

Due to the practices are not performed under conditions of maximum asepsis, diseases such as hepatitis and HIV tetanus can occur, as well as sub-acute bulbar or urinary infections. Severe blood loss along with poor diet and hereditary diseases can cause severe anaemia. The extirpation of the bulbar area will produce sexual, obstetric and gynecological obstetric complications since this organ has a very heterogeneous functionality. Sexual complications do not necessarily have to be associated with the absence of orgasm because other factors are involved, but disparuremia, decreased sexual desire, anorgasmia and sexual sensitivity may occur. Gynecological complications include dysmenorrhea and hematocolpos (Kelly and Hillard, 2015).

### 4.1.3 Genitourinary complications

Genitourinary complications are recurrent urinary tract infections due to the slow and painful emptying of the bladder. Often a dehydration picture is associated, as many women avoid drinking fluids .Obstetric complications are generated at the time of delivery and depends on the degree of mutilation that due to the loss of elasticity due to the formation of keloids and dermoid cysts due to scarring of the skin make it difficult to deliver. In the postpartum haemorrhages due to atony and urinary infections due to retention may occur (Braddy and Files, 2007).

### 4.1.4 Psychological consequences

The psychological consequences are intimately linked to the culture because they are caused by the contradictory feelings induced by the difference of values of the society in which they live and the culture to which they correspond, which causes fear of being rejected by their own people. They do not submit to this practice. In the culture of these women if they have not undergone genital mutilation, they can hardly marry, which will lead to depression and anxiety. It has also been described a specific syndrome called "genitally focused anxiety depression" or what is the same "anxiety-depression syndrome genitally focused", which is characterized by a constant concern of girls or women who have suffered ablation on the state of their genitals and panic to infertility (Utz-Billing & Kentenich,2008). However, these psychological consequences of those women who have migrated to Western countries usually have problems related to the difference of culture of the new country, since genital mutilation is not usually well regarded. This can lead to serious internal conflicts of identity and loyalty to their own culture, experiencing feelings of humiliation, confusion, helplessness, sense of family betrayal and shame (Nour, 2004).

## 4.2 A complex reality

Female genital mutilation is legitimized through beliefs that justify its maintenance. In order to dismantle the practice of FGM/C, it is important to evaluate those beliefs that reflect ablation as something positive (Boyle, 2005). FGM/C is believed to be a rite of initiation of girls into adulthood, a step for integration into the community and for the support of the group's social cohesion and identity. These females at the time of marriage are not considered pure if they are not genitally mutilated. However, this argument loses its force when, according to the WHO, the average age to carry out this practice has now been reduced . The reasons for reducing the average age are diverse. Among them, reduce the possible resistance of the girl to mutilation, reduce the traumatic effects and avoid legal reprisals in the countries where FGM/C is considered illegal (Afifi and Won, 2007).

There are also justifications of a sexual nature. This argument focuses on ensuring the control of women's sexuality, so as to ensure their virginity and fidelity, linked to family honor. Moreover, it is also believed that mutilated women are more fertile, and that mutilation improves and facilitates childbirth. Likewise, one of the justifications is for the female to be hygiene as the not mutilated female is considered impure. Due to this reason, in some countries, mutilation is called purification. Furthermore, aesthetic causes are also included, as it is believed that the female genitals is not beautiful (Catania et al, 2007).

FGM/C is not an exclusive practice of the African community, although today it is where it is most widespread. FGM/C is practiced among the Muslim, Christian and Jewish population. Moreover, in the 19th century, mutilation was practiced under medical precepts to cure the supposedly female hysteria. On the other hand, scholars have discovered that some Egyptian mummies of the second millennium before Christ have female genital mutilation, therefore, overthrows the denominator of religion given the polytheistic space in which the Egyptian mummies lived. In fact, although the arguments used for FGM/C practice vary from one society to another, what seems clear is that this practice determines the role of females within their communities. This role places the female in an unequal position inferior to that of men, where the control of female's body and her sexuality constitutes one of the central axes for maintaining the patriarchal power (Hellsten, 2004).

When the practices of female gentile mutilation are considered for the case of Oman, a very complex reality is faced, which deserves an integral approach by the administrations involved. Although in its 2015 publication on FGM/C, UNISEF reported that " evidence suggests that the procedure is being performed" in Oman, not much data is available to estimate the number of Omani females who are at risk of FGM/C every year. In its February issue 2014, the Y magazine in Oman published the Grand Mufti of Oman, Sheikh Ahmed bin Hamad al Khalili response on the question of female Circumcision:

> Circumcision is allowed in Sunnah, and none of the old Ulama (religious legal scholars) have said it was hated, but they have disagreed if it's a must or a preferable Sunnah to do, or allowed to do. They (the hadith) never mount up that it is a must, and it was always mentioned in relation to male circumcision. It could not be described as a crime against women or as a violation of women's rights', but it was clear that the operation must not cause any

damage. What is referred to as FGM is not the practice that the Sunnah talked about. Circumcision is simple and clear to cut a piece of the clitoris without causing any damage, everything that is not this, shouldn't be called circumcision. Therefore whatever the WHO (World Health Organisation) described as circumcision is not accurate as these are bad practices of those unable to perform proper circumcision. Therefore, circumcision is not allowed by sharia if it causes damage, this is a rule, and if it was medically proven by well trusted doctors that circumcising women will cause damage, it should be banned based on the no harm rule of the sharia. (Ginn, 2014)

Contrary to the Grand Mufti of Oman, Sheikh Ahmed bin Hamad al Khalili response on the question of female circumcision is published on the Ministry of Endowment and Religious Affairs. He states on the English page which is titled *Birth Rites and Rituals* that "Female circumcision is prohibited by law"("Birth rites and rituals", 2018). However, nothing is mentioned about the prohibition of female circumcision on the Ministry's original page in Arabic.

On the one hand, international organizations and researchers are advocating elimination of FGM/C practices due to the health care consequences associated with them, whereas on the other hand, the practice is widely pursued in Oman without even getting officially reported. From the analysis of these practices in terms of their association with the culture, tradition and beliefs of women in Oman, a different perspective on the pursuit of these practices is revealed. It was initially anticipated that due to the rise of modernism and educational level for women in this country, the practices are more likely to be already on the path of elimination. However, the perspective of women about its significance tells a different story.

This research has explored the various dimensions surrounding the acceptance of FGM/C practices. Also, the cases of African and other countries have been studied for reporting various social and health care implications associated with the practices of FGM/C. The rationale behind acceptance of such practices have been elaborated to give a perspective on the situation in Oman, where a high number of families are still practicing FGM/C at home owing to their firm beliefs and perceptions associated with the practice.

Majority of research advocates that FGM/C is a health problem. It indicates violent and painful treatment of females. Because of this reason, to reach a resolution, the use of criminal law as a sanctioning mechanism cannot be dissociated from adequate information and prevention work through organizations such as schools, social services, health professionals, intercultural mediators and educators. However, for the case of Oman, analysis shows that no direct laws have been implemented to term these practices prohibited due to the nature of cultural and social sensitivity associated with the matter. It is noted that women are the most anxious to circumcise their daughters in Oman as they perceive it as a recommendable practice for young girls. On record, only limited information may be available for the presence of such practices and it may appear that FGM/C is rarely practiced; however, due to cultural acceptance, the practice may be more common than it has been reported .

# Bibliography-Section One

Abdalla, R. (1982). Sisters in affliction: Circumcision and infibulation of women in Africa. London: Zed Press.

Abdulcadir, J., Margairaz, C., Boulvain, M., & Irion, O. (2011). Care of women with female genital mutilation/cutting. Swiss Med Wkly, 140(8), w13137.

Abdulcadir, J., Rodriguez, M. I., & Say, L. (2015). Research gaps in the care of women with female genital mutilation: an analysis. BJOG: An International Journal of Obstetrics &Gynaecology, 122(3), 294-303.

Afifi, M., & Von Bothmer, M. (2007). Egyptian women's attitudes and beliefs about female genital cutting and its association with childhood maltreatment. Nursing & health sciences, 9(4), 270-276.

Alavi, R. (2003). Female genital mutilation: a capabilities approach.

Al-Hinai, H. (2014). Female Genital Mutilation in the Sultanate of Oman. Retrieved online via: http://www. stopfgmmideast. org/wp-content/uploads/2014/01/habiba-al-hinai-female-genital-mutilation-in-thesultanate-of-oman1. pdf 26 Stop FGM in the Middle East. Oman. http://www. stopfgmmideast. org/countries/oman.

Alice, B. (2011). Listening to African voices. Female Genital Mutilation/Cutting among Immigrants in Hamburg: Knowledge, Attitudes and Practice, Plan International Deutschland e. V., Hamburg.

Al Mukrashi, F. (2015). Omani students arrested in UK over genital mutilation request. Retrieved from http://gulfnews. com/news/gulf/oman/omani-students-arrested-in-uk-over-genital-mutilation-request-1.1525729

Andro, A., Cambois, E., & Lesclingand, M. (2014). Long-term consequences of female genital mutilation in a European context: self perceived health of FGM women compared to non-FGM women. Social science & medicine, 106, 177-184.).

Assembly, U. G. (1979). Convention on the elimination of all forms of discrimination against women. Retrieved April, 20, 2006.

Bansal, S., Breckwoldt, M., O'Brien Green, S., & Mbugua, S. (2013). Female genital mutilation: Information for health-care professionals working in Ireland 2nd edition.

Baron, E. M., & Denmark, F. L. (2006). An exploration of female genital mutilation. Annals of the New York Academy of Sciences, 1087(1), 339-355.

Barrett, L. (2014). Physical Integrity and Human Rights. The SAGE Handbook of Human Rights: Two Volume Set, 145.

Behrendt, A. (2011). Listening to African Voices: Female Genital Mutilation, Cutting Among Immigrants in Hamburg: Knowledge, Attitudes and Practice. Plan.

Behrendt, A., & Moritz, S. (2005). Posttraumatic stress disorder and memory problems after female genital mutilation. American Journal of Psychiatry, 162(5), 1000-1002.

Berg, R. C., & Denison, E. (2012). Does female genital mutilation/cutting (FGM/C) affect women's sexual functioning? A systematic review of the sexual consequences of FGM/C. Sexuality research and social policy, 9(1), 41-56.

Berg, R. C., & Denison, E. (2013). A tradition in transition: factors perpetuating and hindering the continuance of female genital mutilation/cutting (FGM/C) summarized in a systematic review. Health care for women international, 34(10), 837-859.

Berg, R. C., & Underland, V. (2013). The obstetric consequences of female genital mutilation/cutting: a systematic review and meta-analysis. Obstetrics and Gynecology International, 2013.

Blanchfield, L., & Browne, M. A. (2013). The United Nations Educational, Scientific, and Cultural Organization (UNESCO). Congressional Research Service.

Birth rites and rituals. (2018). Retrieved from http://www.mara. om/religion-in-oman/modern-day-in-oman/birth-rites-and-rituals/

Boyle, E. H. (2005). Female genital cutting: Cultural conflict in the global community. JHU Press.

Boyle, E. H., Songora, F., & Foss, G. (2001). International discourse and local politics: Anti-female-genital-cutting laws in Egypt, Tanzania, and the United States. Social Problems, 48(4), 524-544.

Braddy, C. M., & Files, J. A. (2007). Female genital mutilation: cultural awareness and clinical considerations. Journal of Midwifery & Women's Health, 52(2), 158-163.

Branco, L. M., Hilary, M. O. E., & Cintra, I. D. P. (2006). Body perception and satisfaction in adolescents and the relationship with their nutritional status. Archives of Clinical Psychiatry. White, L. M., Hilary, M. O. E., & Cintra, I. D. P. (2006). Body perception and satisfaction in adolescents and the relationship with their nutritional status. Archives of Clinical Psychiatry.

Braun, V. (2010). Female genital cosmetic surgery: a critical review of current knowledge and contemporary debates. Journal of Women's Health, 19(7), 1393-1407.

Catania, L., Abdulcadir, O., Puppo, V., Verde, J. B., Abdulcadir, J., & Abdulcadir, D. (2007). Pleasure and orgasm in women with female genital mutilation/cutting (FGM/C). The journal of sexual medicine, 4(6), 1666-1678.

Geraci, D., & Mulders, J. (2016). Female genital mutilation in Syria? An inquiry into the existence of FGM in Syria. Utrecht: Pharos.

Cerejo, D. (2017). Female genital mutilation. Responding to Domestic Violence: Emerging Challenges for Policy, Practice and Research in Europe, 231.

Chandra-Mouli, V., Svanemyr, J., Amin, A., Fogstad, H., Say, L., Girard, F., & Temmerman, M. (2015). Twenty years after International Conference on Population and Development: where are we with adolescent sexual and reproductive health and rights?. Journal of Adolescent Health, 56(1), S1-S6.

Committee on Bioethics. (1998). Female genital mutilation. Pediatrics, 102(1), 153-156.

COUNCIL, O. E. (2008, December). Committee of Ministers. In Decisions adopted at 1043rd DH meeting (pp. 2-4).

Creighton, S., Dear, J., de Campos, C., Williams, L., & Hodes, D. (2015). Multidisciplinary approach to the management of children with female genital mutilation (FGM) or suspected FGM: service description and case series. Retrieved from http://10.1136/bmjopen-2015-010311

Darby, R., & Svoboda, J. S. (2007). A rose by any other name? Rethinking the similarities and differences between male and female genital cutting. Medical anthropology quarterly, 21(3), 301-323.

Dorkenoo, E., & Elworthy, S. (1992). Female Genital Mutilation: Proposals for Change. Minority Rights Group International Report.[Revised]. Minority Rights Group International, London, United Kingdom.

Earp, B. D. (2014). Female genital mutilation (FGM) and male circumcision: Should there be a separate ethical discourse?.

Female Circumcision in Oman. (2005). Retrieved from https://wikileaks.org/plusd/cables/05MUSCAT402_a.html

Female Genital Mutilation/Cutting: A statistical overview and exploration of the dynamics of change. (2013). Retrieved from http://data.unicef.org/wp-content/uploads/2015/12/FGMC_Lo_res_Final_26.pdf

Female Genital Mutilation Part of National Action Plan. (2006). Retrieved from https://wikileaks.org/plusd/cables/06MUSCAT1065_a.html

Friedlander, M. L., Covens, A., Glasspool, R. M., Hilpert, F., Kristensen, G., Kwon, S., ... & Russell, P. (2014). Gynecologic Cancer InterGroup (GCIG) consensus review for mullerian adenosarcoma of the female genital tract. International Journal of Gynecological Cancer, 24(9), S78-S82.

Ghimire, R. (2016). Reproductive, Sexual and Maternal Health of Women in Oman. Retrieved from https://www.researchgate.net/publication/297729999_Conference_Paper_Reproductive_Sexual_and_Maternal_Health_of_Women_in_Oman

Gilbert, L. (2017). Female Genital Mutilation and the Natural Law. The National Catholic Bioethics Quarterly, 17(3), 475-486.

Ginn, K. (2014). The Deepest Cut. Retrieved from https://issuu.com/ytabloid/docs/306

Glasier, A., Gülmezoglu, A. M., Schmid, G. P., Moreno, C. G., & Van Look, P. F. (2006). Sexual and reproductive health: a matter of life and death. The Lancet, 368(9547), 1595-1607.

GSN, W. T., Newsgroup, G. S., & Feed, G. L. (2006). Female genital mutilation and obstetric outcome: WHO collaborative prospective study in six African countries. Lancet, 367(9525), 1835-1841.

Health Systems Profile- Oman. (2006). Retrieved from http://apps.who.int/medicinedocs/documents/s17304e/s17304e.pdf

Hellsten, S. K. (2004). Rationalising circumcision: from tradition to fashion, from public health to individual freedom—critical notes on cultural persistence of the practice of genital mutilation. Journal of Medical Ethics, 30(3), 248-253.

Hicks, E. (2018). Infibulation: female mutilation in islamic Northeastern Africa. Routledge.

Hofstede, G. (2003). Culture's consequences: Comparing values, behaviors, institutions and organizations across nations. Sage publications.

Human Rights Watch Submission to the CEDAW Committee of Oman's Periodic Report for the 68th Session. (2017). Human Rights Watch. Retrieved 5 April 2018, from https://www.hrw.org/news/2017/10/10/human-rights-watch-submission-cedaw-committee-omans-periodic-report-68th-session

Hunter College. Women's and Gender Studies Collective. (2015). Women's Realities, Women's Choices: An Introduction to Women's and Gender Studies. Oxford University Press.

Isenberg, L. M., & Elting, L. M. (1976). The Consumer's Guide to Successful Surgery. New York: St. Martin's.

Isenberg, S., & Elting, L. M. (1976). A guide to sexual surgery. Cosmopolitan, 181(5), 104-108.

Jaffer, Y., Afifi, M., Al Ajmi, F., & Alouhaishi, K. (2006). Knowledge, attitudes and practices of secondary-school pupils in Oman: II. Reproductive health. Eastern Mediterranean Health Journal, 12(1-2), 50-60. Retrieved from http://applications.emro.who.int/emhj/1201_2/12_1-2_2006_50_60.pdf?ua=1

Johnsdotter, S. (2003). Somali women in Western exile: reassessing female circumcision in the light of Islamic teachings. Journal of Muslim Minority Affairs, 23(2), 361-373.

Johnsdotter, S. (2009). The FGM legislation implemented: Experiences from Sweden. Malmo University, Sweden, available online at www. Uv.es/CEFD/17/Johnsdotter pdf.

Kaplan, A., Hechavarría, S., Martín, M., & Bonhoure, I. (2011). Health consequences of female genital mutilation/cutting in the Gambia, evidence into action. Reproductive health, 8(1), 26.

Kelly, E. A., & Hillard, P. J. A. (2005). Female genital mutilation. Topics in Obstetrics & Gynecology, 25(26), 1-5.

Khaja, K., Barkdull, C., Augustine, M., & Cunningham, D. (2009). Female genital cutting: African women speak out. International Social Work, 52(6), 727-741.

Kutscher, J. (2011). Towards a solution concerning female genital mutilation? An approach from within according to Islamic legal opinions. Scripta Instituti Donneriani Aboensis, 23, 216-236. Retrieved from https://journal.fi/scripta/article/view/67389

Leveraging Education to End Female Genital Mutilation/Cutting Worldwide. (2016). Retrieved from https://www.icrw.org/wp-content/uploads/2016/12/ICRW-WGF-Leveraging-Education-to-End-FGMC-Worldwide-November-2016-FINAL.pdf

Lightfoot-Klein, H. (1989). Prisoners of ritual (p. 167). Haworth Press.

Mackie, G. (2000). Female genital cutting: the beginning of the end. Female" circumcision" in Africa: culture, controversy, and change. Boulder, Colorado, Lynne Rienner, 253-282.

Martingo, C. (2009): Or cut two female genitalia in Portugal

Meeting a Circumciser: "Men suffer from it" – In Salalah facing up against FGM is almost impossible. (2013). Retrieved from https://stopfgmmiddleeast.wordpress.com/2013/12/06/meeting-a-circumciser-men-suffer-from-it-in-salalah-facing-up-against-fgm-is-almost-impossible/

Meyer, E. (2015). Designing Women: The Definition of Woman in the Convention on the Elimination of All Forms of Discrimination against Women. Chi. J. Int'l L., 16, 553.

Middelburg, A., & Balta, A. (2016). Female Genital Mutilation/ Cutting as a Ground for Asylum in Europe. International Journal of Refugee Law, 28(3), 416-452.

Mitike, G., &Deressa, W. (2009). Prevalence and associated factors of female genital mutilation among Somali refugees in eastern Ethiopia: a cross-sectional study. BMC public health, 9(1), 264.

M'jamtu-Sie, N. (2007). The impact of culture and tradition on attitudes to health in Sierra Leone. Journal of Hospital Librarianship, 6(4), 93-107.

Momoh, C. (2017). Female genital mutilation. In The Social Context of Birth (pp. 143-158). Routledge.

Nour, N. M. (2008). Female genital cutting: a persisting practice. Reviews in Obstetrics and Gynecology, 1(3), 135.

Nowak, M. (2012). Torture: Perspective from UN Special, Rapporteur on Torture and Other Cruel, Inhuman or Degrading Treatment. NTU L. Rev., 7, 465.

Oberreiter, J. A. (2008). A cut for lifetime. The case of female genital mutilation among the community of Guinea Bissau in Lisbon (Doctoral dissertation, Dissertação de Mestrado em Direitos Humanos e Democratização. Faculdade de Direito da Universidade Nova Lisboa).

OHCHR, U., UNDP, U., UNESCO, U., UNHCR, U., & UNIFEM, W. (2008). Eliminating female genital mutilation: an interagency statement. Geneva: WHO, 22-70.

Oman. (2013). Retrieved from http://orchidproject.org/wp-content/uploads/2013/11/Oman-Final.pdf

Oman. (2014). Retrieved from http://spring-forward.unwomen. org/en/countries/oman

Oman. (2018). Genderindex.org. Retrieved 5 April 2018, from https://www.genderindex.org/country/oma

Oman, S., Oman, S., & profile, V. (2012). FGM / Female Circumcision in Oman. Shawawioman.blogspot.com. Retrieved 5 April 2018, from http://shawawioman.blogspot.com/2012/01/fgm-female-circumcision-in-oman.html

Onuh, S. O., Igberase, G. O., Umeora, J. O., Okogbenin, S. A., Otoide, V. O., & Gharoro, E. P. (2006). Female genital mutilation: knowledge, attitude and practice among nurses. Journal of the National Medical Association, 98(3), 409.

Rahman, A., &Toubia, N. (Eds.). (2000). Female genital mutilation: A practical guide to worldwide laws & policies. Zed Books.

Reisel, D., & Creighton, S. M. (2015). Long term health consequences of Female Genital Mutilation (FGM). Maturitas, 80(1), 48-51.

Robinett, P. (2006). The Rape of Innocence: One Woman's Story of Female Genital Mutilation in the USA. Aesculapius Press.

Roth, R. (2013). Female Genital Mutilation. Violence Against Girls and Women: International Perspectives [2 volumes]: International Perspectives, 115.

Sajó, A. (2013). Human rights with modesty: the problem of universalism. Springer.

Saul, B., Kinley, D., & Mowbray, J. (2014). The international covenant on economic, social and cultural rights: commentary, cases, and materials. OUP Oxford.

Shell-Duncan, B., &Hernlund, Y. (Eds.). (2000). Female" circumcision" in Africa: culture, controversy, and change. Lynne Rienner Publishers.

Sipsma, H. L., Chen, P. G., Ofori-Atta, A., Ilozumba, U. O., Karfo, K., & Bradley, E. H. (2012). Female genital cutting: current practices and beliefs in western Africa. Bulletin of the World Health Organization, 90, 120-127.

Skaine, R. (2005). Female genital mutilation: Legal, cultural and medical issues.

Tag-Eldin, M. A., Gadallah, M. A., Al-Tayeb, M. N., Abdel-Aty, M., Mansour, E., &Sallem, M. (2008). Prevalence of female genital cutting among Egyptian girls. Bulletin of the World Health Organization, 86, 269-274.

Toubia, N. (1995). Female genital mutilation. Women's Rights, Human Rights: International Feminist Perspectives, 224-37.

UNESCO (2002)Universal Declaration on Cultural Diversity

UNICEF. (2005). Female genital mutilation/cutting: a statistical exploration 2005. Unicef.

UNICEF. (2016). Female genital mutilation/cutting: a global concern. New York: UNICEF, 1-4.

Utz-Billing, I., & Kentenich, H. (2008). Female genital mutilation: an injury, physical and mental harm. Journal of Psychosomatic Obstetrics & Gynecology, 29(4), 225-229.

Van Gennep, Arnold (1960) The Rites of Passage. Chicago: University of Chicago Press.Marcusán, A. K. Introduction to Female Genital Mutilation from an Anthropological Perspective.

Wadesango, N., Rembe, S., & Chabaya, O. (2011). Violation of women's rights by harmful traditional practices. The Anthropologist, 13(2), 121-129.

Wangila, M. N. (2015). Female Circumcision: The Interplay of Religion, Culture and Gender in Kenya (Women from the Margins). Orbis Books.

Weiss, H. A., Quigley, M. A., & Hayes, R. J. (2000). Male circumcision and risk of HIV infection in sub-Saharan Africa: a systematic review and meta-analysis. Aids, 14(15), 2361-2370.

Wettig, H. (2014). In Oman more than 80% of women could be mutilated – Results of a two-week field trip. Retrieved from https://stopfgmmiddleeast.wordpress.com/2014/01/31/in-oman-more-than-80-of-women-could-be-mutilated-results-of-a-two-week-field-trip/

Whitehorn, J., Ayonrinde, O., & Maingay, S. (2002). Female genital mutilation: cultural and psychological implications. Sexual and Relationship Therapy, 17(2), 161-170.

Wille, B. (2014). Female Genital Mutilation in Yemen (p. 27). USA: Human Rights Watch.

Wollman, L. (1973). Female circumcision. Journal of American Society of Psychosomatic Dentistry and Medicine, 12, 130-1. Yount, K. (2002). Like mother, like daughter? Female genital cutting in Minia, Egypt. Journal of Health and Social Behavior, 43, 336-358.

World Health Organization (2001) Female Genital Mutilation: A Student's Manual. Department of Gender and Women Health, WHO, Geneva.

World Health Organization. (2001). Management of pregnancy, childbirth and the postpartum period in the presence of female genital mutilation: report of a WHO technical consultation, Geneva, 15-17 October 1997.

World Health Organization. (2011). Progress in scale-up of male circumcision for HIV prevention in Eastern and Southern Africa: focus on service delivery-2011 revised.

World Health Organization. (2015). Health in 2015: from MDGs, millennium development goals to SDGs, sustainable development goals.

Xiong, B. Female Genital Mutilation: Rituals Around the Globe and its Horrifying Effects.

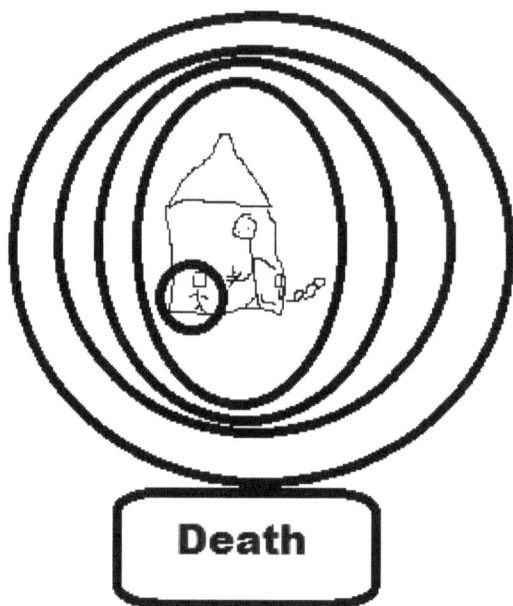

Death

# SECTION TWO

## THE PREVALENCE OF

## FGM/C PRACTICE IN OMAN

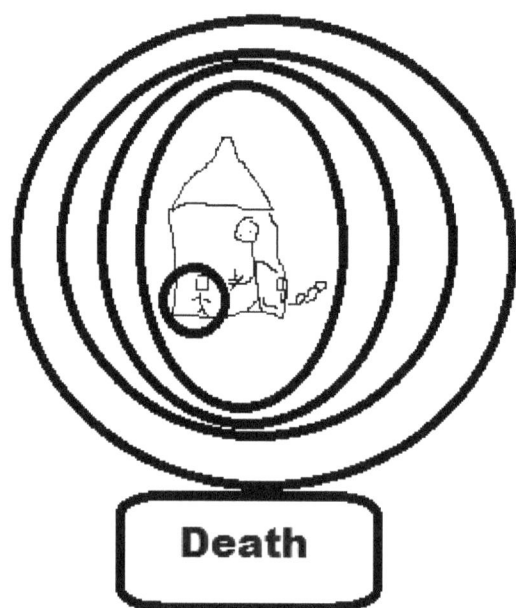

**Death**

# Table of Contents-Section Two

# Chapter One : Introduction

## 1.1 Preface

Female genital mutilation/cutting (FGM/C) is a form of gender-based violence that is prevalent across a number of countries, communities and ethnic groups worldwide. Viewed in the western world as a violation of human rights, FGM/C is a practice that is deeply-rooted in the traditions and beliefs of many patriarchal cultures across Africa and into the Middle East and Asia. It is a misogynistic practice that contributes to gender inequalities and results in huge amounts of emotional and physical suffering. The cutting, scraping, piercing, removing and sewing of the female genitalia results in serious health consequences and is typically performed on children under the age of ten.

## 1.2 Limitations of Existing Data

To date, the majority of the data available on the topic of FGM/C originates from studies conducted in Africa. While there has been research published regarding FGM/C in the Middle East, the data is sparse. This is particularly true in the case of Oman, a predominantly Muslim country located on the east coast of the Arabian Peninsula. The World Health Organization (WHO) and the United Nations Children's Emergency

Fund (UNICEF) do not typically include Oman in their lists of countries where FGM/C is known to be practiced. To our knowledge, the only study that has examined the prevalence of FGM/C within Oman is a 2014 survey of 100 women living in the capital city of Muscat (Al Hinai, 2014). In this population, 78% of participants self-reported themselves as having been cut (Al Hinai, 2014). It is important to note that the prevalence of FGM/C is likely to vary regionally as well as between ethnic, religious and socioeconomic groups. Unfortunately data examining these factors as they relate to the prevalence of FGM/C in Oman is extremely limited. There is a considerable need for high-quality research investigating the practice of FGM/C across populations and regions of Oman.

## 1.3 Statement of Purpose

The aim of this study is twofold:

**1-To investigate and report upon the prevalence of FGM/C in Oman;**

**2-To determine which attributes among the surveyed population are associated with the decision to cut their own daughter(s).**

Equipped with this new information, recommendations may be made that target the practice of FGM/C in Oman with the intention of increasing awareness and education. Opening up the discourse regarding FGM/C and its prevalence in Omani society may pave the way for the formation of support groups for victims of FGM/C and as well as community programs. Insights gained from this study may also be useful in the creation of new policies at the institutional level condemning FGM/C. The eventual eradication of this horrific and harmful practice is the ultimate goal.

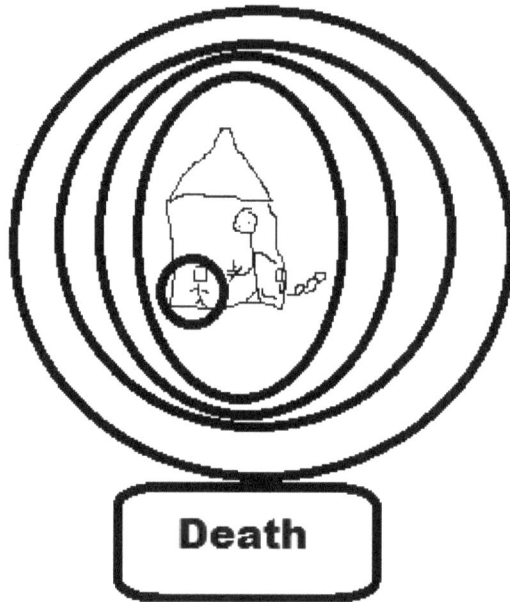

Death

# Chapter Two : Review of the Literature

## 2.1 Definition of female genital mutilation/cutting (FGM/C)

The term "female genital mutilation" refers to all procedures involving the partial or total removal of the external genitalia, or any damage inflicted to the female genitalia for non-medical reasons (WHO, UNICEF, UNFPA, 1997). The practice of female genital mutilation, or FGM, can also be referred to colloquially as "cutting." For the purposes of this project, our research team adopted the definition and typologies set forth by the WHO/UNICEF/UNFPA in their Joint Statement from 1997, which was subsequently updated in 2008.

### 2.1.1 Types of FGM/C

The WHO, UNICEF and UNFPA (2008) categorize FGM/C according to the following criteria:

**Type I**–Partial or total removal of the clitoris and/or the prepuce

**Type II**–Partial or total removal of the clitoris and the labia minora, with or without excision of the labia majora (excision)

**Type III**–Narrowing of the vaginal orifice with creation of a covering seal by cutting and appositioning

113

the labia minora and/or the labia majora, with or without excision of the clitoris (infibulation)

**Type IV**–All other harmful procedures to the female genitalia for non-medical purposes, for example: pricking, piercing, incising, scraping and cauterization.

It is estimated that 90% of mutilation occurrences worldwide fall under the category of Type I, II or IV while 10% of cases are Type III (WHO & Pan American Health Organization, 2012). Type III is generally considered to be the most severe of the four categories and it is important to note that the relatively small percentage of 10% equates to approximately 8 million women globally. In Africa alone, approximately 130 million female children have been subjected to genital mutilation and 3 million per year are at risk (WHO & Pan American Health Organization, 2012).

### 2.1.2. Effects of FGM/C on health outcomes

One of the major issues with FGM/C is that it is often performed using unsanitary methods. Procedures are generally carried out with rudimentary tools and without anesthetic. The tools used may not be not sterilized or the same instrument may have been used for excisions on other individuals (which could lead to the spread of diseases such as HIV). Among the instruments used are knives, pieces of glass and sticks.

### 2.1.2.1 Short-term consequences

During and immediately following the procedure, many girls enter a state of shock induced by the extreme pain, psychological trauma and exhaustion from screaming. The procedure can result in death through severe bleeding leading to haemorrhagic shock, or as a result of infection and septicaemia. Other immediate medical complications include ulceration of the genital region, injury to adjacent tissues and urine retention (Berg, Underland, Odgaard-Jensen, Fretheim & Vist, 2014).

### 2.1.2.2 Long-term consequences

In the months and years following FGM/C, girls and women may experience serious problems during menstruation, urination, intercourse, pregnancy and childbirth. Although the scientific research addressing the psychological consequences of FGM/C is limited, some studies have found an increased likelihood of fear of sexual intercourse, post-traumatic stress disorder, anxiety, depression. As a victim of FGM/C matures, her sexuality will also be affected. A decrease and/or absence of sensitivity and sexual pleasure, dyspareunia, anorgasmia and fear of sexual relations may occur (Berg et al., 2014). Vaginal penetration through injured and scarred genital tissue may be difficult or impossible, with rupture of the tissue, causing further bleeding and severe pain (Onuh, 2006).

## 2.2 Belief system surrounding FGM/C

FGM/C is a tradition based on misconceptions. It is a practice that corresponds to the archaic beliefs regarding a woman's place in the community. FGM/C is a social problem based on gender discrimination and stigmatization, rooted in asymmetries of power, reflecting one of the many forms of violence against women–physical, psychological, sexual–and with dire consequences for the health, education and empowerment of children, youth and women victims of the practice (Baron and Denmark, 2006).

Female genital mutilation is a very old practice, likely originating even before the appearance of monotheistic religions. Neither its origin nor its place of birth is completely clear. Some historians have established that in ancient Egypt, excision was practised between 5000 and 6000 BC during the time of the Pharaohs. Some scholars have been able to find mutilated sex organs in bodies of mummified women (Cerejo, 2017). The specific name "infibulation" has its origin during ancient Rome and comes from the word "fibula" which was the brooch with which the Roman women's togas were closed. The interpretation that could be that infibulation is the closing of the feminine genital organs, perhaps to force a young woman to remain a virgin before marriage.

In these social structures that are based on unbalanced power relations and in the inequality between the sexes, women occupy a position of inferiority while men exercise a function of dominion over sexuality, autonomy, and their lives. The woman, according to an archaic patriarchal concept, would be the depository of the family honour, which would explain the prejudices about their promiscuity and the need of control over their bodies. The social and family pressure suffered by girls is of such magnitude that most do not even conceive of being able to refuse to undergo mutilation. Those who try are marginalized, rejected and isolated from their group. In most cases, little or no training and information about their sexuality makes the victims completely ignorant of the true magnitude of the trauma they will suffer. They only know the physical consequences of mutilation and such vexation "has always existed for women".

There is a belief that the female genitals are "unclean" so that only through extirpation can they be purified. In some communities, women who have not suffered genital mutilation are considered dirty and are forbidden from handling food or water, as they are supposed to intoxicate or poison them. It is also based on the idea that only man has the right to enjoy sexual pleasure. In addition, it is founded on traditional beliefs, values and attitudes. Depending on the country, culture or region, it is believed that this practice increases fertility and facilitates childbirth, improves the level of hygiene and makes the female genitals more beautiful. They believe that they are releasing a woman from a dangerous organ, as in some cultures, it is believed that the clitoris will render men sterile if their genitals come into contact, or the newborn will die (Behrendt, 2011).

## 2.3 FGM/C: A violation of human rights

FGM/C is a violation of human rights. The practice of FGM/C is a brutal act of violence that directly affects the physical and psychological integrity of the victim. Undoubtedly, as established in Article 3 of the European Convention on Human Rights, the mutilation of genital organs of girls and young women constitutes "inhuman and degrading" treatment (Duffy, 1983). In addition to violating the basic rights of children and women, FGM/C also violates the sexual and reproductive rights of these girls and women, as it deprives them of making decisions about their own bodies. There are several international organizations, such as the Orchid Project, that intend to work towards the eradication of FGM/C, both from the point of view of an implementation of public policies, prevention, and sensitization of communities, as well as criminalization of the practice.

## 2.4 Factors associated with FGM/C across multiple populations

### 2.4.1 Age

FGM/C is usually practiced on children between the ages of 4 and 12 years old. However, in some cultures the procedure happens at birth, before marriage, or during the first pregnancy, and is usually celebrated by the family and community, marking the transition to adulthood. In addition, it is important to note that some women are excised more than once during their lifetime, such as after childbirth (very common in infibulation communities), which is called "reinfibulation" (Rushwan, 2000). However, according to UNICEF, the average age at which girls are subjected to FGM/C is falling in some countries (UNICEF, 2013). It is attributed to a possible consequence of the adoption of national legislation that prohibits it, which has encouraged families to carry out their practice at an earlier age, so that it is easier to hide from the authorities.

### 2.4.2 Place of residence

It has been previously observed that populations living in rural areas have higher prevalence rates of FGM/C than populations living in urban areas (Setegn, Lakew & Deribe, 2016; Kandala & Komba, 2015). However it is possible that shift will soon be observed where rates rise in urban zones, possibly due to migratory tendencies towards urban areas.

### 2.4.3 Education and socioeconomic status

It has been shown that the higher the educational level of women within a community, the less likely they are to subject their daughters to FGM/C (Alkhalaileh, Hayford, Norris & Gallo, 2018; Chikhungu & Madise, 2015; Van Rossem, Meekers & Gage, 2015). It has also been shown that in households whose wealth level is higher, the FGM/C index is lower than in poor households. In countries such as Chad, Benin, Kenya and Mauritania it was found that 60% of the households where FGM/C had been practiced on women in the family were poor households (UNICEF, 2005).

### 2.4.4 Religion

Contrary to popular belief, no religion prescribes FGM/C. It is practiced by Muslim groups, by certain Christian and Jewish groups, as well as by the followers of some animistic religions. It is a cultural tradition, not religious. The practice of FGM/C predates Christianity and Islam, although many believe that this is a religious obligation (Behrendt, 2011). Although there is a theological branch of Islam that supports it, the Sunna type, the Quran does not include any text that requires the ablation of the external genital organs of women. It is important to note that al-Azhar Supreme Council of Islamic Research, the highest religious authority in Egypt, made a statement declaring that the practice of FGM/C has no basis in core Islamic law or any of its partial provisions and that it is detrimental and should not be practiced.

## 2.4 Prevalence and current perceptions of FGM/C in Africa and the Middle East

According to the WHO, the practice of FGM/C has been documented in 29 African countries (WHO, 2008). The Orchid Project, a UK-based charity that advocates against FGM/C, reported that among women 15 to 49 years-old, the highest rates of FGM/C are in Egypt (87%), Sudan (87%), Mali (89%), Sierra Leone (90%), Djibouti (93%), Guinea (97%) and Somalia (98%) (Richards, 2017). The practice of FGM/C has also been documented in South and South-east Asia, the Middle East and in Colombia, however no national statistics are available.

## 2.5 Prevalence and current perceptions of FGM/C in Oman

In 2006, Jaffer et al. conducted a valuable study that investigated the social attitudes of Omani adolescents. The study revealed that 80% of both girls and boys who participated in the project approved of FGM/C practices, and thought of them as "necessary and important." Hence, it is not merely a matter of gender inequality in Oman but of an inclination in the whole culture towards acceptance of these practices.

### 2.5.1 Legality of FGM/C in Oman

In Oman, no direct laws have been implemented to declare FGM/C prohibited. However, the practice was officially banned in both government and private health facilities in Oman in January 2001.

### 2.5.2 Availability of Oman-specific data

There is no unified state registry of the number of mutilated women and girls living in Oman's territory. Presently the only Oman-specific data available was released in a 2014 report of survey findings from 100 women living in Muscat, the country's capital city (Al Hinai, 2014). In this population, 78% of participants self-reported themselves as having been cut (Al Hinai, 2014). This data is valuable but not without limitations. In addition to the study's small sample size, and perhaps more importantly, the participants were surveyed in the largest and most prosperous city in Oman. Muscat is relatively progressive when compared to the rest of the country and it may be reasonable to assume that FGM/C is less common in more liberal, urban areas. While nationwide reports would be ground-breaking, data from other regions of the country would also be extremely valuable.

# Chapter Three : Study Design and Data Collection Methods

## 3.1 Study Population

Participants surveyed for the purpose of this project were Arabic-speaking females living in the ad-Dakhiliya province of Oman. In total, 200 women were surveyed. An overview of the study population can be found below in section 4.1 (Population Demographics).

## 3.2 Study Questionnaire

The study questionnaire and the Informed Consent Form were translated into Arabic from English and were administered by an Arabic-speaking research team member who is a Family and Community Medical Doctor . A document outlining the questions from the questionnaire can be found in Appendix **A1** and **A2**. A copy of the Informed Consent Form can be found in Appendix **B1** and **B2**.

## 3.3 Data Collection Methods

The survey was conducted between October and December of 2017 in a public government medical center in ad-Dakhiliya, Oman. Informed consent was obtained from each participant prior to the administration of the study survey. To complete the questionnaire, a Senior Specialist (MRCGP) in Family and Community Medicine, interviewed each patient verbally. Participants did not undergo a physical clinical examination at the time of the survey.

# Chapter Four: Results and Discussion

### 4.1 Population Demographics

Study participants were primarily between the ages of 19 and 45 years old. The vast majority of the population (94%) hailed from the province of ad-Dakhiliyah. Almost the entire study population (97.5%) self-reported their ethnicity as being Omani. Only 7% of the women surveyed stated that they were currently single, whereas 96% reported themselves as married. Participants came from various educational backgrounds with 5.5% having received either a primary school education or no education, 40.5% having attained a secondary school education and 50.5% having obtained a diploma or completed university-level training. Among participants, 44% were currently employed while the remainder reported themselves as either students or "housewives."

**Table 1** - Patient demographics of 200 women surveyed in a public government medical center in ad-Dakhiliya, Oman between October and December 2017

Abbreviation - FGM: female genital mutilation
Total N=200 unless otherwise specified

| Participant demographics | Total, n (%) |
|---|---|
| *Age, years* | |
| 15-18 | 0 (0.0) |
| 19-25 | 37 (18.5) |
| 26-35 | 88 (44.0) |
| 36-45 | 49 (24.5) |
| 46-55 | 2 (1.0) |
| 56-65 | 1 (0.5) |
| 65+ | 1 (0.5) |
| Not reported | 22 (11.0) |

| Marital status | |
|---|---|
| Single | 7 (3.5) |
| Married | 192 (96.0) |
| Divorced | 1 (0.5) |
| Widow | 0 (0.0) |
| Not reported | 0 (0.0) |

| *Ethnicity* | |
|---|---|
| Omani | 195 (97.5) |
| African | 2 (1.0) |
| Asian | 2 (1.0) |
| Ajmi | 0 (0.0) |
| Baluchi | 0 (0.0) |
| Not reported | 1 (0.5) |

| Province of origin | |
| --- | --- |
| Ad-Dakhiliyah | 188 (94.0) |
| Ad-Dhahirah | 3 (1.5) |
| Muscat Governorate | 1 (0.5) |
| Al-Wusta | 2 (1.0) |
| Ash-Sharqiyah | 2 (1.0) |
| Al-Batinah | 3 (1.5) |
| Not reported | 1 (0.5) |

| *Level of education attained* | |
| --- | --- |
| Illiterate | 3 (1.5) |
| Primary education | 8 (4.0) |
| Preparatory education | 7 (3.5) |
| Secondary education | 81 (40.5) |
| Diploma | 25 (12.5) |
| Bachelor Degree | 72 (36.0) |
| Higher education | 4 (2.0) |
| Not reported | 0 (0.0) |

| Occupation | |
|---|---|
| House wife | 107 (53.5) |
| Student | 4 (2.0) |
| Employed | 88 (44.0) |
| Retired | 0 (0.0) |
| Not reported | 1 (0.5) |

## 4.2 FGM/C among the surveyed population

95.5% of the women surveyed for the purpose of this study self-reported themselves as having been cut in their lifetimes. Among the 191 women who had undergone genital mutilation, 65% stated they had been subjected to Type I mutilation, 3.1% stated they had been subjected to Type II while 57.1% of the women stated "I don't know." 28.5% of the women were mutilated at one year or less of age, whereas 20% were cut between the ages of two years and ten years old. 47.0% of the women surveyed were uncertain of the age at which they were cut. The vast majority (94.3%) of the women stated that they had been cut by a "local woman" and the women reported that in most cases the mutilation was carried out at home (91.6%).

**Table 2** - FGM/C among 200 women surveyed in a public government medical center in ad-Dakhiliya, Oman between October and December 2017

Abbreviation - FGM: female genital mutilation
Total N= 200 unless otherwise specified

| Participant characteristics relating to FGM | Total, n (%) |
|---|---|
| *Undergone FGM* | |
| Yes | 191 (95.5) |
| No | 5 (2.5) |
| "I don't know" | 0 (0.0) |
| Not reported | 4 (2.0) |

| Type of FGM, (n=191) | |
|---|---|
| Type I | 65 (34.0) |
| Type II | 6 (3.1) |
| Type III | 0 (0.0) |
| "I don't know" | 109 (57.1) |
| Not reported | 11 (5.8) |

| Age at time of mutilation, (n=191) | |
|---|---|
| At birth | 16 (8.0) |
| 1 year | 41 (20.5) |
| 2 years | 8 (4.0) |
| 3 years | 8 (4.0) |
| 4 years | 8 (4.0) |
| 5 years | 5 (2.5) |
| 6 years | 2 (1.0) |
| 7 years | 4 (2.0) |
| 8 years | 2 (1.0) |
| 9 years | 1 (0.5) |

| Age at time of mutilation, (n=191) | |
|---|---|
| 10 years | 2 (1.0) |
| "I don't know" | 94 (47.0) |
| Not reported | 0 (0.0) |
| *Location where mutilation was performed, (n=191)* | |
| At home | 175 (91.6) |
| At a clinic | 7 (3.7) |
| "I don't know" | 2 (1.0) |
| Not reported | 7 (3.7) |

| Person who performed the mutilation, (n=191) | |
|---|---|
| Specialized nurse | 7 (3.7) |
| A local woman | 180 (94.3) |
| "I don't know" | 2 (1.0) |
| Not reported | 2 (1.0) |

## 4.3 Participant perceptions and opinions regarding FGM

Across the 200 women who participated in this study, 85.0% reported that they agree with FGM/C as a practice. "Religious reasons" were found to be the predominant factors on which the opinions were based among 72.5% of participants, whereas 11.0% stated "cultural reasons." 68.5% of the women surveyed reported having female children of their own and 86.0% had had their daughter(s) cut or planned to have their daughter(s) cut in the future. When sub-grouped based on if they themselves had been subjected to FGM/C, 92.4% of women who had been cut planned to have their daughters mutilated, or had had their daughters already cut. No woman who had not been mutilated herself, stated that she planned to have, or already had, her daughter(s) cut.

**Table 3** - Perceptions and general opinions of FGM/C among 200 women surveyed in a public government medical center in ad-Dakhiliya, Oman between October and December 2017

Abbreviation - FGM: female genital mutilation

Total N= 200  unless otherwise specified

| Participant opinions regarding FGM | Total, n (%) |
|---|---|
| *General opinion of FGM as a practice* | |
| "I agree" | 170 (85.0) |
| "I do not agree" | 19 (9.5) |
| "I don't know" | 3 (1.5) |
| Not reported | 8 (4.0) |

| Basis of opinion regarding FGM | |
| --- | --- |
| Religious reasons | 145 (72.5) |
| Cultural reasons | 22 (11.0) |
| Family reasons | 0 (0.0) |
| Religious&cultural reasons | 7 (3.5) |
| Cultural and family reasons | 0 (0.0) |
| Religious and family reasons | 0 (0.0) |
| "I don't know" | 1 (0.5) |
| Not reported | 25 (12.5) |

| Daughter(s) of their own | |
|---|---|
| Yes | 137 (68.5) |
| No | 60 (30.0) |
| Not reported | 3 (1.5) |
| **Plan to - or have had - FGM performed on daughter(s)** | |
| Yes | 172 (86.0) |
| No | 18 (9.0) |
| "I don't know" | 1 (0.5) |
| Not reported | 9 (4.5) |

## 4.4 Association between various population characteristics and their decision to cut their daughter(s)

By conducting a chi-square test of independence, it was revealed that variables significantly associated with the decision to cut their daughter(s) were: having undergone FGM/C themselves ($X^2 = 38.60$, p-value<0.05), level of education attained by the study participant ($X^2 = 23.93$, p-value p-value<0.05) and the occupation/employment status of the study participant ($X^2 = 14.05$, p-value<0.05). Age of the participant was not significantly associated with the decision to have FGM/C performed on their daughter(s) ($X^2 = 0.65$, p-value = 0.72). Analyses investigating marital status, ethnicity and home province were not conducted due to the high level of homogeneity among participants (i.e. the under-dispersal of values).

**Table 4** - Associations between various patient demographics of 200 women surveyed in ad-Dakhiliya,
Oman between October and December 2017 and their
decisions to have their own daughters undergo FGM/C

Abbreviation - FGM: female genital mutilation
* = considered statistically significant

| Decision to cut their daughter(s) | | | | | |
|---|---|---|---|---|---|
| Participant demographics | **Yes** | | **No** | | $^2$ | p-value |
| | N | % | N | % | | |
| **Age, (n=169)** | | | | | | |
| ≤35 years | 107 | 69.0 | 11 | 78.6 | | |
| 36-55 years | 46 | 29.7 | 3 | 21.4 | 0.65 | 0.72 |
| ≥55 years | 2 | 1.3 | 0 | 0.0 | | |
| **Undergone FGM themselves, (n=188)** | | | | | | |
| Yes | 170 | 100.0 | 14 | 77.8 | | |
| | | | | | 38.60 | <0.05* |
| No | 0 | 0 | 4 | 22.2 | | |

| Level of education (n=190) | | | | | |
|---|---|---|---|---|---|
| ≤ Primary education | 10 | 5.8 | 1 | 5.6 | |
| Preparatory or secondary education | 108 | 62.8 | 1 | 5.6 | 23.93 | <0.05* |
| ≥ Bachelor degree | 54 | 31.4 | 16 | 88.9 | |
| **Occupation, (n=190)** | | | | | |
| House wife | 101 | 58.7 | 2 | 11.8 | |
| Student | 3 | 1.7 | 1 | 5.9 | 14.05 | <0.05* |
| Employed | 68 | 39.5 | 14 | 82.4 | |

# Chapter Five: Conclusion and Future Directions

Results from this study indicate that FGM/C is highly prevalent and also widely accepted among Omani females. In total, 95.5% of the study population reported that they had undergone FGM/C in their lifetime. Perhaps not surprisingly, many of the women (56.1%) were uncertain as to what type of FGM/C had been performed on them. Of particular interest is that 72.5% of the women surveyed stated "religious reasons" for the belief they hold regarding FGM/C. This is a highly disturbing finding. As previously mentioned, FGM/C is not prescribed by any religion and has no place in Islam according to the al-Azhar Supreme Council of Islamic Research.

Age was not associated with participants' decisions to have their daughter(s) undergo FGM/C, demonstrating that the general perception regarding FGM/C is independent of age group. However women who obtained a university-level education reported more frequently that they did not plan to, or had not already, cut their daughters when compared to participants who had not received a university-level education. This finding is consistent with the current literature (Alkhalaileh et al., 2018; Chikhungu & Madise, 2015; Van Rossem et al., 2015).

Another finding that supports a trend previously reported in the literature (Van Rossem et al., 2015) is that women who were employed were significantly more likely to report that they did not plan to, or had not already, cut their daughters when compared to women who self-reported themselves as students or "housewives." Lastly, it was observed that within the population, women who had not been cut themselves were significantly more likely to answer that they had no intention of, or had not already, cut their daughters when compared to women who had been subjected to FGM/C.

It is important to note that, although it is hopeful to see that some women had no plans to have their daughters undergo FGM/C, the vast majority of the surveyed population did. In total, 86.0% of women reported that they intended to, or had already had, their daughters cut. This is highly troubling and alarming finding as it suggests that many young girls are at risk of being cut in present-day Omani society.

It is also important to note that there were several limitations of our study. Firstly, the recruitment location allowed for only a small snapshot of Omani culture, and may not have been representative of the entire Omani population. As an example, only women seeking care from a specific region of Oman were recruited to participate in this project. In addition, the study population was uniform with regard to their home province. Future projects should be undertaken nationwide, in both rural and urban settings, with larger sample sizes and more diverse populations.

## 5.1 RECOMMENDATIONS

Countless generations of women have been subjected to FGM/C worldwide. However, a shift towards the abolition of the practice is possible with the right backing and supports. The following recommendations were created primarily with the goal of education in mind. A wide body of global research show that offering education on FGM/C "is a central issue in the elimination of FGM" ("Country Profile : FGM in Tanzania", 2013). Hence, there is a need for FGM/C to be integrated into the education system in schools and into the Healthcare higher education programs. Medical education in Oman was commenced in 1986. Between 1993 to 2005, 876 students graduated as Medical specialists ("Health Systems Profile- Oman", 2006). However, FGM/C was not, and is not, included in the study-programs.Creating focused educational programs is suggested to address the issue of FGM/C in Oman at its grass-root levels with the help of trained medical practitioners.

By informing populations that FGM/C is harmful, dangerous, unnecessary and not supported by many religious leaders, it is conceivable that future generations may be liberated from the violating, barbaric practice of FGM/C.

### 5.1.1 Formally ban FGM/C at the governmental level (Ministry of Health)

With FGM/C formally banned, it is hopeful that hospital and clinic staff will no longer be permitted to turn a blind eye to the mutilations that occur on their premises.

### 5.1.2 Request the support of religious leaders

Women in this study reported "religious reasons" as being the most common rationale for the beliefs they hold regarding FGM/C. By educating the followings of various religious groups that FGM/C is not an element of their teachings, it is possible that families and communities will be less inclined to practice cutting.

### 5.1.3 Conduct a national study

The highly diverse rural and urban areas of Oman create

a major barrier in studying the spread of FGM/C in the country. The southern province of Dhofar is considered anecdotally to be the most conservative region of Oman and therefore it may be reasonable to suspect that FGM/C is more commonplace there than in urban areas. A nationwide study would be highly beneficial.

### 5.1.4 Provide education in maternity wards

Healthcare practitioners in clinics and hospitals such as nurses and doctors may be influential groups to target. Enlisting their help in educating families and new mothers may be highly beneficial.

### 5.1.5 Create educational materials

The creation of pamphlets and posters may be a method of educating the public by hand them out in doctors' offices and hospitals.

### 5.1.6 Form support groups

The formation of groups within communities would be beneficial in a number of ways. By introducing the concept that FGM/C is unnecessary and harmful to smalls groups of men and women, it is possible that the belief system may shift favourably. By providing support to women who have undergone FGM/C, they may feel empowered.

**Do not plan to cut daughter(s)**

**Plan to cut daughter(s)**

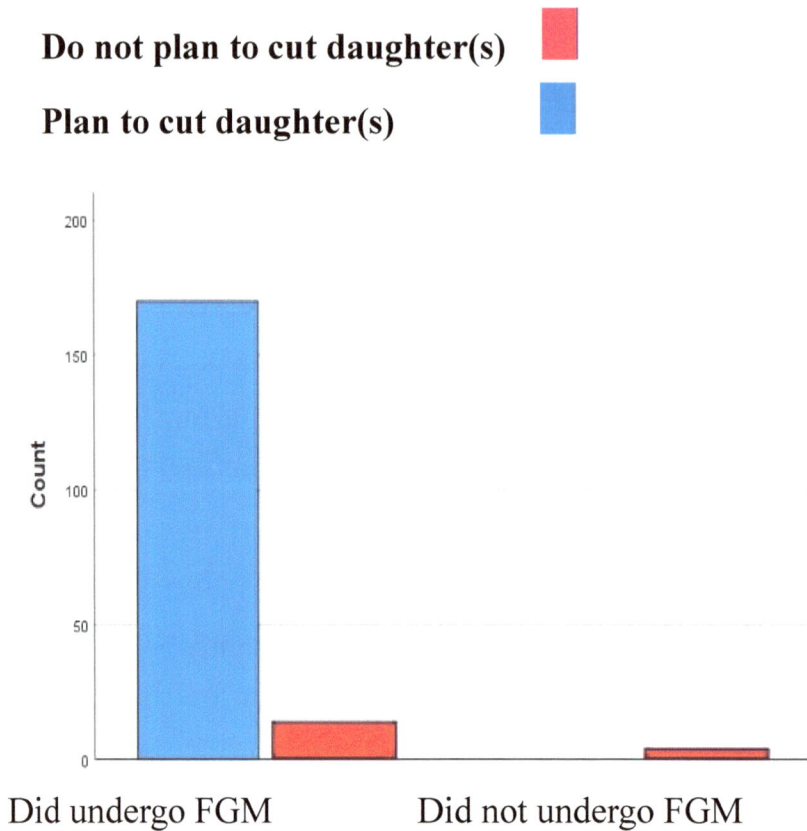

Did undergo FGM                    Did not undergo FGM

**Figure 1** - Bar graph depicting the number of women who plan to - or have had - their own daughter(s) cut, categorized on the basis of whether or not they themselves had undergone FGM/C as girls  **(n=188)**

**Do not plan to cut daughter(s)** ■

**Plan to cut daughter(s)** ■

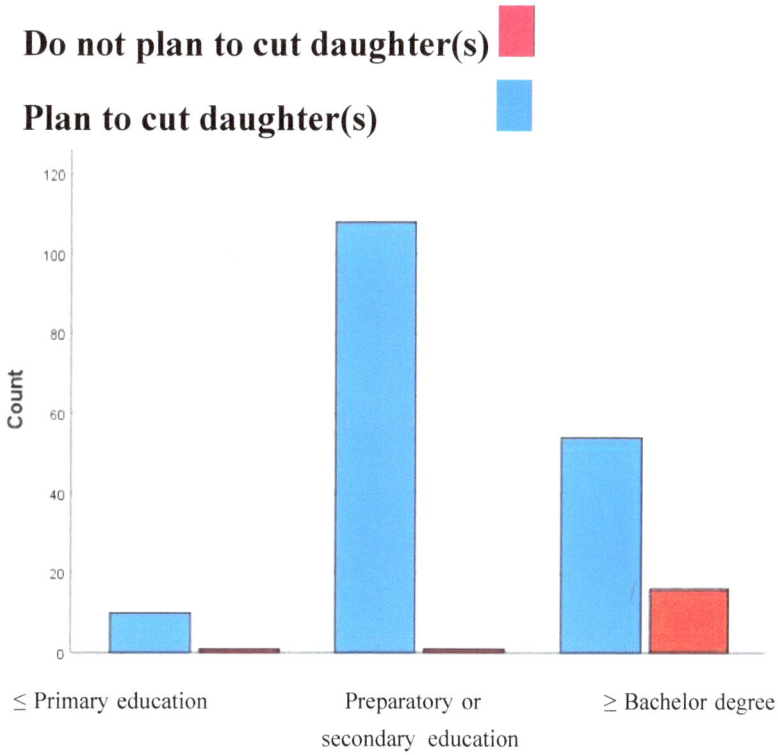

**Figure 2** - Bar graph depicting the number of women who plan to - or have had - their own daughter(s) cut, categorized on the basis of the level of education attained by the study participant **(n=190)**

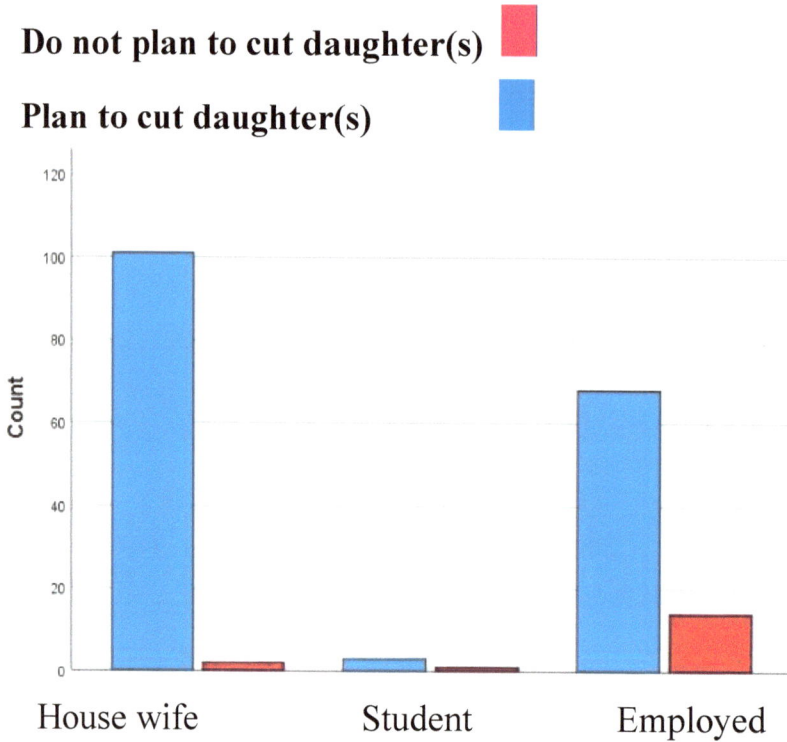

**Figure 3** - Bar graph depicting the number of women who plan to - or have had - their own daughter(s) cut, categorized on the basis of the occupation/employment status of the study participant **(n=190)**

## 5.1.7 Include modules on FGM/C in the medical training at Sultan Qaboos University

Educating the future generation of physicians and nurses is of utmost importance. By introducing the concept early and teaching methods to deal with families who plan to mutilate their daughters or who have already, the young healthcare workers will be prepared.

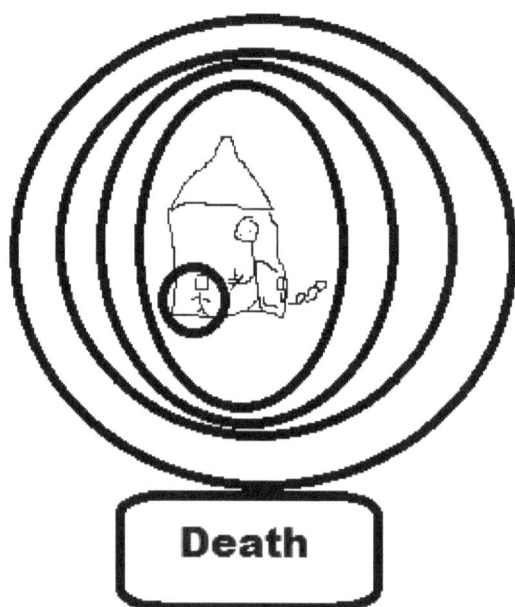

Death

156

# Bibliography-Section Two

Al-Hinai, H. (2014). Female Genital Mutilation in the Sultanate of Oman. Retrieved online via: http://www.stopfgmmideast.org/wp-content/uploads/2014/01/habiba-al-hinai-female-genital-mutilation-in-thesultanate-of-oman1.pdf 26 Stop FGM in the Middle East. Oman. http://www.stopfgmmideast.org/countries/oman.

Alkhalaileh, D., Hayford, S. R., Norris, A. H., & Gallo, M. F. (2018). Prevalence and attitudes on female genital mutilation/cutting in Egypt since criminalisation in 2008. Culture, Health & Sexuality, 20(2), 173-182.

Baron, E. M., & Denmark, F. L. (2006). An exploration of female genital mutilation. Annals of the New York Academy of Sciences, 1087(1), 339-355.

Berg, R. C., Underland, V., Odgaard-Jensen, J., Fretheim, A., & Vist, G. E. (2014). Effects of female genital cutting on physical health outcomes: A systematic review and meta-analysis. BMJ Open, 4(11), e006316.

Behrendt, A. (2011). Listening to African Voices: Female Genital Mutilation, Cutting Among Immigrants in Hamburg: Knowledge, Attitudes and Practice. Hamburg: Plan Germany.

Cerejo, D. (2017). Female Genital Mutilation. Responding to Domestic Violence: Emerging Challenges for Policy, Practice and Research in Europe, 231.

Chikhungu, L. C., & Madise, N. J. (2015). Trends and protective factors of female genital mutilation in Burkina Faso: 1999 to 2010. International Journal for Equity in Health, 14(1), 42.

Duffy, P. J. (1983). Article 3 of the European Convention on Human Rights. Int'l & Comp. LQ, 32, 316.

Country Profile : FGM in Tanzania. (2013). Retrieved from https://www.28toomany.org/static/media/uploads/Country%20Research%20and%20Resources/Tanzania/tanzania_country_profile_v1_(december_2013).pdf

Health Systems Profile- Oman. (2006). Retrieved from http://apps.who.int/medicinedocs/documents/s17304e/s17304e.pdf

Jaffer, Y.A., Afifi, M., Al Ajmi, F. & Al Ouhaishi, K.(2006). Knowledge, attitudes and practices of secondary-school pupils in Oman: II. Reproductive health.

Kandala, N. B., & Komba, P. N. (2015). Geographic variation of female genital mutilation and legal enforcement in sub-saharan Africa: A case study of Senegal. The American Journal of Tropical Medicine and Hygiene, 92(4), 838-847.

Onuh, S. O., Igberase, G. O., Umeora, J. O., Okogbenin, S. A., Otoide, V. O., & Gharoro, E. P. (2006). Female genital mutilation: Knowledge, attitude and practice among nurses. Journal of the National Medical Association, 98(3), 409.

Richards, J. (2017). FGC around the world. London: The Orchid Project.

Rushwan, H. (2000). Female genital mutilation (FGM) management during pregnancy, childbirth and the postpartum period. International Journal of Gynecology & Obstetrics, 70(1), 99-104.

Setegn, T., Lakew, Y., & Deribe, K. (2016). Geographic variation and factors associated with female genital mutilation among reproductive age women in Ethiopia:A national population based survey. PloS One, 11(1), e0145329.

United Nations Children's Fund (2005). Female genital mutilation/cutting: A statistical exploration. New York: UNICEF.

United Nations Children's Fund (2016). Female Genital Mutilation/Cutting: A global concern. New York: UNICEF.

United Nations Children's Fund (2013). Female Genital Mutilation/Cutting: A statistical overview and exploration of the dynamics of change. New York: UNICEF.

Van Rossem, R., Meekers, D., & Gage, A. J. (2015). Women's position and attitudes towards female genital mutilation in Egypt: A secondary analysis of the Egypt demographic and health surveys, 1995-2014. BMC Public Health, 15(1), 874.

World Health Organization & Pan American Health Organization. (2012). Understanding and addressing violence against women: Femicide. Geneva: World Health Organization.

World Health Organization, UNICEF & United Nations Population Fund. (1997). Female genital mutilation:A joint WHO/UNICEF/UNFPA statement. Geneva: World Health Organization.

World Health Organization. (2008). Eliminating female genital mutilation: An interagency statement - OHCHR, UNAIDS, UNDP, UNECA, UNESCO, UNFPA, UNHCR, UNICEF, UNIFEM, WHO. Geneva: World Health Organization.

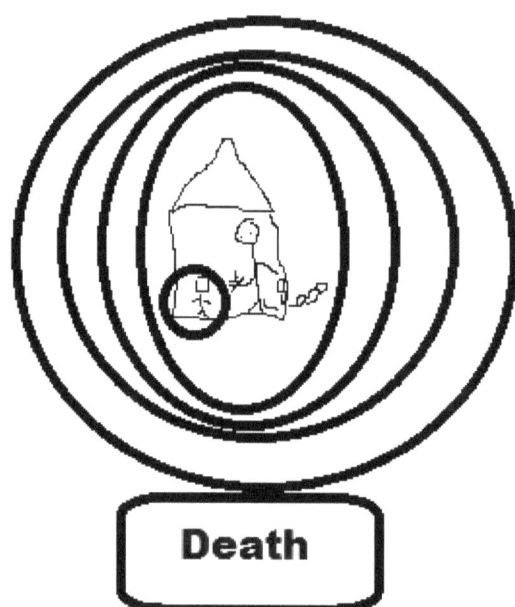

Death

# Appendix

## List of Tables and Graphs

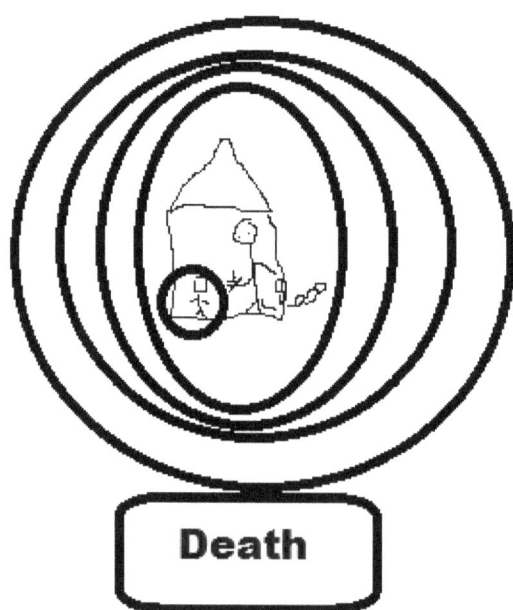

Death

**1.Study questionnaire in English(Appendix A1)**

**Age: How old you are?**

Between 15-18, Between 19-25, Between 26-35, Between 36-45, Between 46-55, Between 56-65, More than 65

**What is your Marital Status?**

Single,       Married,      Divorced,    Widow

**Origins: From which Ethnicity you are?**

Omani,       African,      Asian,     Ajmi,     Balouchi

**Area: From which Province in Oman you are?**

Ad-Dakhiliyah, Ad-Dhahirah, The capital area Muscat, Al-Wusta, Ash-Sharqiyah, Al-Batinah

**Education: What is the level of your Education ?**

No education,       Primary education ,
Preparatory education,  Secondary education,
Diploma, Bachelor Degree,  Higher education

**Career: What is your Occupation?**

House wife,  Student,     Employed,  Retired

**Have you been circumcised ?**

Yes            No

**If you have been circumcised, what type it is?**

Type I — Partial or total removal of the clitoris and/ or the prepuce (clitoridectomy)

Type II — Partial or total removal of the clitoris and the labia minora

Type III — Narrowing of the vaginal orifice with creation of a covering seal by cutting and appositioning the labia minora and/or the labia majora

I don't know

**If you have been circumcised, how old were you?**

At birth, 1 , 2 , 3 , 4 , 5 , 6, 7 , 8 , 9 , 10 , I don't know

**If you have been circumcised, where was it?**

At home                           in a clinic

**If you have been circumcised, who performed the act?**

A specialized nurse  -A traditional health practitioner

**What is your opinion about circumcision?**

I agree                                    I don't agree


**If you agree on circumcision, explain the reason/s?**

Religious reasons          Cultural reasons
Family pressure


**Do you have daughters?**

Yes          No


**If you have a daughter, have you circumcised her or  will you circumcise her?**

Yes          No

## 2. Informed Consent Form in English (Appendix B1)

**Title:** Female Genital Mutilation in Oman

**Investigators:**

*Azza al-Kharousi* (A Senior Specialist
in Family and Community Medicine, Oman).

*Hoda Thabet* ( Ph.D in Comparative Literature,
Iceland)

You are being asked to participate in a research study.

**Purpose:** This study surveys the Omani female. The aim is to understand the spread of Female Genital Mutilation in Oman and the reasons for practising Female Genital Mutilation as well as the personal and social affects of Female Genital Mutilation.

**Procedures:** You will be asked to answer a questionnaire on Female Genital Mutilation in Oman. You will be asked questions about your personal experience and opinions.

**Risks:** It is anticipated that there will be minimal risk, if any, for participants. The survey questions focus on personal experience in Female Genital Mutilation; thus, some participants may experience negative feelings, such as stress, when sharing their stories. In reflecting on your experiences, painful memories may surface. You are encouraged to not answer any question that feels uncomfortable.

**Benefits:** Your participation in this research project will help generate a better understanding about the spread of Female Genital Mutilation in Oman.

**Confidentiality:** Data will be collected through answering the questionnaire. Findings will be reported anonymously without any identifying information which could link participants of the study.

**Your rights:** Your participation is voluntary. You may choose not to participate in this study. If you consent to participate, you may skip any question that you would prefer not to answer in the survey.

By signing this form, you are indicating that you have read and understood the study as it has been described here. You consent to participate in this research study

**Participant's signature:** _____

**Date:** _____

**Investigator's signature:** _____

**Date:** _____

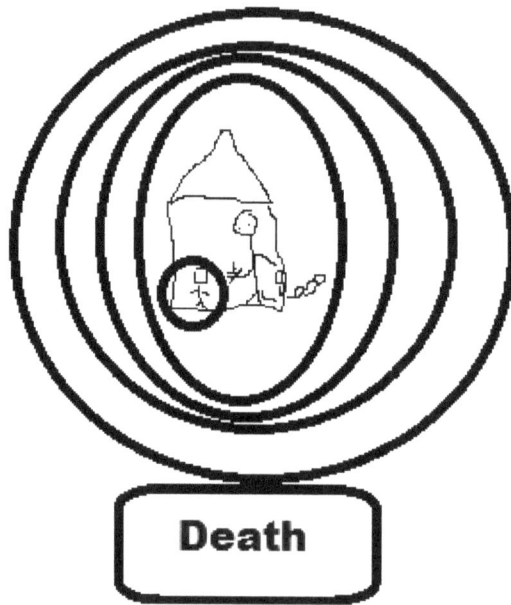

Death

*3.Study questionnaire in Arabic(Appendix A2)*

*4.Informed Consent Form in Arabic(Appendix B2)*

1

عنوان البحث العلمي: **ختان الأنثى في سلطنة عمان**

الباحثات:

**عزة الخروصي** (اخصائي أول طب أسرة ومجتمع ـ سلطنة عمان)

**هدى ثابت** (دكتورة في الأدب المقارن ـ أيسلندة)

قد طلب منك المشاركة في هذا البحث العلمي

**الهدف:** يختص هذا البحث بالأنثى العمانية. الهدف هو معرفة مدى انتشار ظاهرة ختان الأنثى في سلطنة عمان ودراسة أسباب ختان الأنثى والآثار الناجمة عنها على المستوى الفردي والإجتماعي

**الأسلوب:** سيطلب منك الإجابة على استبيان حول ختان الأنثى في سلطنة عمان. ستسألين في هذا الاستبيان أسئلة عن تجربتك وارائك الشخصية في هذا الخصوص

**المخاطر:** من المتوقع وجود مخاطر قليلة جدا للمشاركات ، هذا إن وجدت هذه المخاطر. تركز أسئلة الاستبيان على التجربة الشخصية حول ختان الأنثى. ولهذا، قد تشعر بعض المشاركات بأحاسيس سلبية ، كالتوتر مثلا ، عند مشاركتهن لتجاربهن الشخصية. فعندما تفكرين مليا في تجاربك قد تطفو بعض الأحاسيس المؤلمة على السطح. ولكننا نحثك على أن لا تجيبي على أي سؤال لا تشعرين بالإرتياح في الإجابة عليه

**الفائدة:** عند مشاركتك في هذه الدراسة فإنك ستساهمين في تطوير قاعدتنا المعرفية حول مدى شيوع ظاهرة ختان الأنثى في سلطنة عمان

**السرية:** ستجمع البيانات من خلال توزيع اسئلة الاستبيان على المشاركات. وستنشر النتائج دون ذكر أسماء المشاركات او أي معلومات يمكنها أن تدل على شخصيات المشاركات

**حقوقك:** مشاركتك تطوعية. يمكنك اختيار عدم المشاركة في هذا البحث. لو وافقت على المشاركة، يمكنك حذف أي سؤال تفضلين عدم الإجابة عليه في الاستبيان.

بتوقيعك لهذه الإستمارة، أنت تؤكدين بأنك قد قرأت وفهمت جيدا هذه الدراسة كما وصفت لك هنا. وأنك توافقين على المشاركة في هذا البحث العلمي

توقيع المشترك:

التاريخ :

توقيع الباحث:

التاريخ:

2

استبيان

<u>العمر</u>

بين 15 و 18 - بين 19 و 25 - بين 26 و 35 - بين 36 و 45 - بين 46 و 55 - بين 56 و 65 - أكثر من 65

<u>الحالة الإجتماعية</u>

عزباء - متزوجة - مطلقة - أرملة

<u>من أصول</u>

عمانية - أفريقية - آسوية - عجمية - بلوشية

<u>من المنطقة</u>

الداخلية - الظاهرة - العاصمة - الوسطى - الشرقية - الباطنة

<u>الحالة الدراسية</u>

غير متعلمة - الإبتدائية - الإعدادية - الثانوية - دبلوم - بكالوريوس - دراسات عليا

<u>الحالة الوظيفية</u>

ربة منزل - طالبة - موظفة - متقاعدة

<u>هل أنت مختونة؟</u>

نعم - لا

<u>لو كنت مختونة فهل هي ختان</u>

سطحي من الدرجة الأولى (إزالة جزء أو كل البظر) - متوسط من الدرجة الثانية (إزالة البظر مع الشفرين الصغيرين) - شديد من الدرجة الثالثة (يتضمّن إزالة الشفرين الكبيرين ثم تقطيب وخياطة الجُرح ) - لا أعرف

<u>لو كنت مختونة، فكم كان عمرك</u>

عند الولادة - 1 - 2 - 3 - 4 - 5 - 6 - 7 - 8 - 9 - 10 - لا أعرف

<u>لو كنت مختونة، فأين ختنت؟</u>

في مركز صحي - في البيت

<u>لو كنت مختونة، فمن ختنتك؟</u>

ممرضة متخصصة - إمرأة من عامة الناس تمتهن ختان الانثى (داية)

<u>ما رأيك في ختان الأنثى؟</u>

أوافق - لا أوافق

<u>إذا كنت توافقين على ختان الأنثى، فلماذا؟</u>

أسباب دينية - عادات وتقاليد - ضغط الأسرة

<u>هل عندك أطفال من البنات؟</u>

نعم - لا

<u>لو عندك أطفال بنات، هل ختنت بناتك (هل ستختنين بناتك)؟</u>

نعم - لا

www.ingramcontent.com/pod-product-compliance
Lightning Source LLC
Chambersburg PA
CBHW060812270326
41929CB00002B/11